*Winning Strategies for
Nursing Managers*

Winning Strategies for

Nursing Managers

Joan G. O'Leary, R.N., Ed. D. ✓
Associate Professor, College of Nursing,
Villanova University, Villanova, Pennsylvania

President, O'Leary and Associates, Inc.,
Wayne, Pennsylvania

Sharon Tarrant Wendelgass,
R.N., M.S.N., C.C.R.N.
Nursing Supervisor, Critical Care Module,
The Bryn Mawr Hospital, Bryn Mawr, Pennsylvania

Helen Eckman Zimmerman, R.N., M.S.N.
Nursing Manager, 4th Floor Medicine, University Hospital,
The Milton S. Hershey Medical Center,
The Pennsylvania State University, Hershey, Pennsylvania

J.B. LIPPINCOTT COMPANY
Philadelphia
London   Mexico City   New York
St. Louis   São Paulo   Sydney

Acquisitions Editor: Paul R. Hill
Manuscript Editor: Tina Rebane
Design Director: Tracy Baldwin
Design Coordinator: Earl Gerhart
Designer: Katharine Nichols
Production Supervisor: J. Corey Gray
Production Coordinator: Charlene Catlett Squibb
Compositor: General Graphic Services
Printer/Binder: Philips Offset Co., Inc.

Library of Congress Cataloging-in-Publication Data

O'Leary, Joan G.
  Winning strategies for nursing managers.

  Includes bibliographies.
  1. Nursing service administration. I. Wendelgass,
Sharon Tarrant. II. Zimmerman, Helen Eckman.
III. Title.
  [DNLM: 1. Administrative Personnel. 2. Nursing,
Supervisory—methods. WY 105 045 w]
  RT89.038 1986   362.1′73′068   86-2725
  ISBN 0-397-54541-X

6 5 4 3 2 1

*This book is dedicated to
Dick, Jim, and Loren.*

Acknowledgments

We want to specifically acknowledge the following contributors to this book:

O'Leary and Associates, Inc., (215-688-5752), who contributed the section on patient classification systems

Nancy Voss Coleman, who contributed the section on quality assurance

Dr. Rita Sellers, who contributed the section on collective bargaining

Marilee Warner Mohr, who contributed the nursing philosophy

Steve Shribe, who contributed the Clinical Ladder concept

Linda Goldberg, who was one of the initial writers

Villanova University College of Nursing, which brought us all together.

Contents

Introduction

There was once a Registered Nurse, named Fran, who had been caring for patients for three years. Her patients regarded her as being very competent, and the Doctors relied on her judgment and decision-making abilities. She was regarded by her Head Nurse and by her peers as a "good nurse." But somehow, Fran wasn't satisfied. Why? In the future, she wanted to be a *Nurse Manager*. She wanted to be a *Successful Nurse Manager*.

Fran's quest took her to California, to Arizona, to Pennsylvania. She read a great deal and attended management programs when possible. She spoke with many Directors of Nursing, Nurse Recruiters, and Head Nurses. Her search took her to Community Hospitals, to Community Health Centers, and even to Complex Health Science Centers.

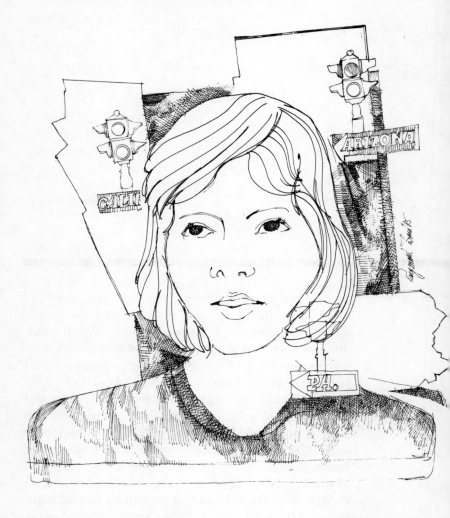

In her travels, Fran always asked the following
questions:

Do you understand yourself in your job?
Do you know the management principles?

Have you been able to apply these principles to the management arena?

As Fran met with and questioned Nurse Managers, she heard some of the Head Nurses say, "Sure, I know who I am, but no one else does . . . ." The nursing units where these Head Nurses worked were in total chaos. Fran also asked these Head Nurses if they knew Management Principles . . . . "What Management Principles?" they would ask. "Why, I barely get through each day." Somehow, these poor managers knew little of themselves and most had no background in management. Their subordinates were frustrated and their bosses were waiting for them to retire.

Fran found other managers. They appeared comfortable with themselves. Their units were well run and their staff motivated. The patients received the best of care, and the Doctors were happy. She asked these successful managers if they had been able to apply management principles to practice. These people said, "Yes! Once you know yourself and what makes a good manager, you can apply these principles and achieve success."

Fran pondered, "Why has this happened to nursing?" Then she thought, "All nurse managers have been nurses much longer than they have been managers. Consequently, the transition from nurse to manager really can be extremely difficult." Over the past three years, she had come to realize that many of those people who were poor nurse managers may have been excellent clinical nurses. They had received preparation to become just that—clinical nurses. So, it wasn't really their fault. It took years to become a nurse, but in the hospital setting a nurse could become a nurse manager overnight.

When Fran moved to the Philadelphia area, she decided that she wanted the experience of working for a tough manager. The Nurse Recruiter, upon hearing Fran's request, smiled and merely stated, "Ms. Herrick is the toughest manager we have. Her floor has a forty percent turnover. Nobody wants to work for her on 5 West . . . ."

When Fran began to work for Ms. Herrick, she noticed that Ms. Herrick always arrived at work on time. Ms. Herrick did tell Fran that she had gained fifty pounds since she took the job of manager twenty years ago. Ms. Herrick rarely smiled, and she was anxiously looking forward to collecting her pension in two more years. Fran noticed that whenever a member of the staff requested a change, Ms. Herrick would shrug her shoulders and say that she would write a memo. After more suggestions from the staff member, Ms. Herrick would finally suggest that perhaps he or she would be happier on another unit.

Two years passed, and the tough Ms. Herrick retired. Throughout this two-year period, Fran learned a great deal from her management courses, readings, and observations. Her management potential was clearly evident throughout her interviews for Ms. Herrick's position. There was little surprise on the part of the medical or nursing staff when Fran was appointed Nurse Manager of 5 West.

Within one and a half years, 5 West had evolved into one of the most efficient and productive units in the hospital. One day, the Director of Nursing called Fran into her office and asked, "How do you do so well?" Fran replied, "I believe in management in three stages." "What is that?" asked the Director. "Well," Fran said:

Stage One is to *understand yourself.*

Stage Two is to *know the management principles.*

Stage Three is to *know how to apply these principles to practice.*

"Success," Fran said, "can be accomplished by *utilizing these three stages.*" Because of Fran's success, the Director replied, "I would like you to begin presenting your three stages of management to the other nurse managers at the Management Council Meeting next week.

Stage 1

Who Am I?

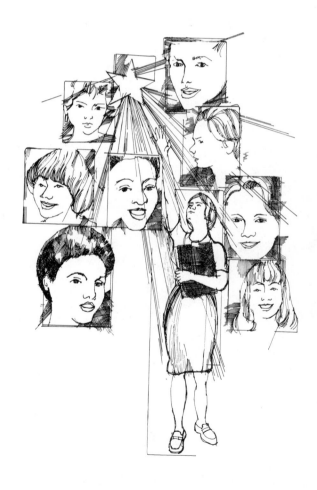

Knowledge of Professional Nursing

For Fran, nursing became a caring process that encompassed a strong scientific base. She learned to apply her knowledge so effectively that she was able to assist individuals in *maintaining wellness* and in *preventing* and *recovering from illness*.

Fran learned to use the *Nursing Process*, and always *assessed her patients*. She gained information not only by *asking questions*, but by *looking* and by *touching* her patients. This *assessment* was always done utilizing a *problem list*—a *list* that she carried with her at all times. The *nursing problems* that Fran considered were the following:

Do you have problems with:

Mobility?

Compliance with your treatment regimen?

Nutrition?

Elimination?

Skin integrity?

Activity?

Pain—alteration in comfort?

Coping needs?

Compliance with medication?

Potential for infection?

Discharge needs?

Educational needs—knowledge of self-care?

Do you need emotional support?

This problem list became Fran's *framework* for *defining nursing diagnoses.* These diagnoses, once identified, became her responsibility to evaluate continually and to resolve. She knew that other Registered Nurses also had this responsibility. She routinely wrote on the Care Plan and included *interventions that she had planned.* . . . that is, those things that had to be done for the patient in order for those problems to be resolved. *These interventions,* then, became *The Nursing Orders.* Every day, when beginning work, she would review *the Problems, the Diagnoses, the Interventions,* and the *Nursing Orders.* The *Nursing Orders changed daily* as her patients progressed. She documented all these changes *on the Patient Care Record,* so that *all* care takers would be aware of the status of the patient.

Fran also kept current *with the Forces Affecting the Profession.* There were many ways she accomplished this task. *Returning to school, joining professional organizations, attending conferences, networking,* and *reading journals* were only a few identified ways through which Fran learned what was really going on in the outside world.

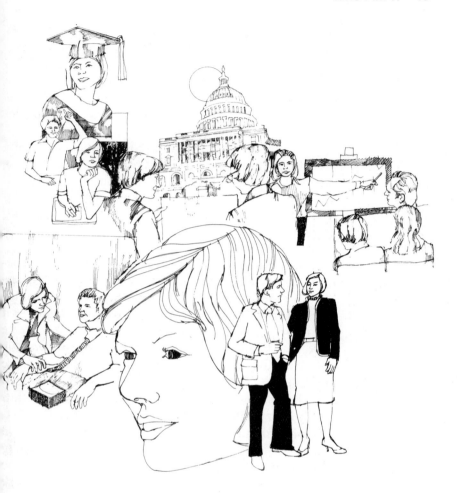

Fran continued *advancing her degrees* in the hopes of achieving substantial leadership in agencies and in the professional organizations. She found a valuable program that broadened and strengthened her base in nursing.

Upon graduation, Fran discovered that there were many graduate programs to prepare nurse managers.

Some of these programs allowed an inspired manager to achieve a Master's Degree in Nursing Administration. She graduated from a Master's Program in Nursing Service Administration. Not only did she become prepared in nursing, she also received a comprehensive base in management theory, budget, nursing research, and nursing theories.

Fran cultivated substantial educational links. She saw that cultivating a good relationship with Directors of Schools of Nursing could benefit both groups. The educators provided a different perspective to the health care environment. They presented a *fresh view,* an *objectivity,* and a *perspective* different from those inside the hospital.

Much was learned by returning to the classroom . . . learning not only from the professors, but also from the students. For Fran, the *networking* that resulted from the socialization of the students over a two-year period lasted a lifetime.

Networking was not new to nursing, but it was new to Fran. She had moved frequently as a child, and after graduating from nursing school she continued that pattern by accepting a staff nurse position in a hospital 300 miles from the school. For this reason, she found *networking* to be both helpful and rewarding. Friendships were not just tossed aside like disposable paper supplies.

Fran developed a system of not only keeping track of other people but of letting other nurses know *where* she was living . . . *what* she was doing presently and hoped to be doing in the near future . . . and *when* she expected to be in their area.

Her system included:

1. Filing name cards
2. Sending a change of address to the schools

from which she had graduated, along with a "Hello" (She was now invited to alumni gatherings.)

3. Attending alumni meetings
4. Attending seminars—and wearing a name tag at those seminars
5. Taking classes—meeting people . . . going out socially with these people
6. Stopping by the school whenever she was in the area to say "Hello" in person

After returning to graduate school, Fran continued the *networking* process she had developed, and this greatly assisted her in her professional development. She began to carry this process even further. When she attended seminars or conferences, she introduced herself to others and left these gatherings knowing at least five new individuals. She *extended her network*. This was sometimes difficult because it meant that she was not always able to sit and talk with "old" friends.

While she was attending school and working at the hospital, Fran continued with her participation on committees. She saw her institution as having to develop corporate relationships with other businesses just to survive. Hospitals and Home Care Agencies were joining forces with other institutions in order to maintain financial viability.

Fran became versed in community health needs. She kept abreast of her surrounding community . . . their needs and wants, and how these needs changed over time. Fran accomplished this by routinely reviewing *newspapers* and *journals*. Reviewing these current articles frequently provided Fran comprehensive insight into current trends. Overall, Fran became responsive to the needs of society at large.

Fran knew she needed "friends in high places." She

found out the names of those who were in the decision-making positions in the federal regulating and legislative agencies. She frequently offered to represent her hospital in presenting nursing concerns to the policy-making people.

She joined the American Nurses Association, which is involved in developing and maintaining the Standards of the Profession. Fran found that the American Nurses Association was also developing and maintaining standards for those in nursing service administration, and she wrote away for and received copies of those standards and shared them with her staff. These standards became the basis for the *Standards of Practice* on her unit. She attended local meetings, which provided her with information and needed networking.

She discovered that the National League for Nursing has a forum called the National Forum for Administrators of Nursing. All Directors of Nursing, and Associate Directors of Nursing, are eligible to join this organization. Her current Director of Nursing was an active member of this forum. Fran found out that this forum is committed to creating a better understanding of the competencies required in administration and works hard at helping education and service achieve common goals. Along with the American Nurses Association, this forum provides a voice in the development of positions on national health policy issues. It provides a vehicle to communicate the view of the nurse executive to the appropriate national agencies. Both organizations, the American Nurses Association and the National League for Nursing, provide leadership opportunities for those interested in nursing management. Fran gained experience and visibility by working on committees, holding an office, and actually publishing papers. These relationships expanded her horizon . . . .

There were many other questions for Fran to ponder . . . Who will actually receive nursing care? Who will pay for this care? What moral and ethical issues are going to confront the nurse at the bedside? What about the role of women and the women's movement? Will nurses continue doing what they are doing now . . . or will the role and function of nursing continue to change?

She addressed and *focused* on these current issues, *stayed abreast of trends,* and became *proactive in the decision-making process . . . not retroactive.*

Visibility—Laying the Groundwork

As Fran thought back over all of the different qualities and behaviors that the successful, competent nurse manager should possess, she felt there was still something missing. Is it enough to answer and to know, "Who am I?" Does the possession of these personality traits, qualities, and behaviors necessarily ensure a successful nurse manager?

Fran thought back to her first nursing position in a large teaching hospital where she had met many dynamic nursing individuals. She could remember the Nurse Manager of her unit, Susan Elsewhere, who had a MSN degree from State University and who seemed very intelligent and very nice. Fran saw her every morning for report and once every two weeks for the unit staff meeting. On occasion, she would see her on the unit for short intervals, but most of the time Ms. Elsewhere was elsewhere at meetings, classes,

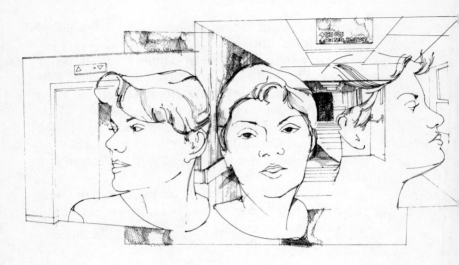

evaluations, or planning days. Fran could remember meeting Ms. Elsewhere's Supervisor twice. This Supervisor also had a MSN degree and she seemed very knowledgeable and very concerned about patient care and nursing needs. As Fran continued to think about her first job, she realized she had never even had an opportunity to meet the Director or Associate Director of Nursing.

These nurse managers with whom she had some contact "seemed" competent and seemed to "know who they were," but Fran wasn't sure that she really knew who they were or that they knew who she was. Is it enough, then, to know oneself and to possess these managerial qualities? Fran concluded that it definitely was not! It is equally important that the nurse manager *be visible!*

If a nurse manager hopes to set the stage for her department, then she must *serve as a role model* and let her objectives and philosophy be known. The mos effective method of accomplishing this is through the following:

Making Rounds—at least every other month on all shifts

Unit Meetings—every two weeks

Meeting individually with staff every six months to discuss personal goals and objectives

Spending time informally with staff

In other words, by *being visible*

By being visible, not only does the staff discover who the nurse manager is and what she hopes to accomplish, but the nurse manager will begin to discover the staff's personal goals and objectives as well as their accomplishments and frustrations. This input can be invaluable in assisting the nurse manager in establishing an environment to ensure quality nursing care.

Leadership Behaviors

To attain the goal of becoming an effective nurse manager, Fran needed to know about *Leadership*. Was there a difference between leadership and management? Yes!

"Managers are persons who hold positions where they are responsible for other workers . . . leaders are persons who, for one reason or another, have a followship" (Stevens, 1980, p. 193). It was going to take time for Fran to develop her *Leadership Style*.

"Leadership," she thought, "involves a social interaction that results in a group following and a group attainment of goals." "Leadership implies activity, movement, getting work done" (Bass, 1981, p. 66). Munson defines leadership as "the ability to handle men so as to achieve the most with the least friction and the greatest cooperation . . . . Leadership is the creative and directive force of morale" (Bass, 1981, p. 9).

Fran continuously *observed* the *leadership role* of the Managers in all of her meetings. She asked herself, *"What traits do these managers possess and what style do they use* in moving the group toward goal attainment?"

Fran observed certain traits that stood out. Managers who "looked the role" were more readily accepted upon first meeting a group. Managers who presented a better appearance than others achieved more success. Those who not only looked the role but who also acted the role were also more readily accepted in a manager's position.

Fran *looked in the mirror* and reached some conclusions about *successful managers:*

Look the role.
Always dress professionally.

Those managers who *talked well,* had a broad *knowledge base,* and kept their *emotions under control* were those who achieved excellence. Those who used *tact* and *diplomacy* elicited the cooperation of groups over those who were abrupt and crude.

Practice public speaking.
Keep learning and asking to expand your knowledge base.

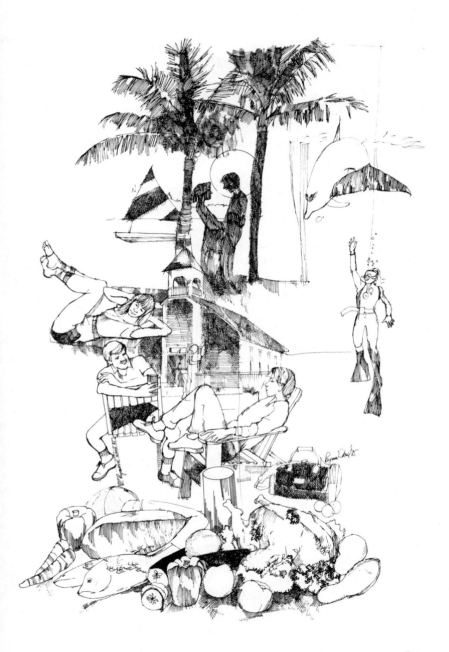

Those managers who *acted alive* and had a high *energy level* appeared to be given additional responsibilities.

> *Act alive, exercise, eat well, get your sleep, keep your weight down,* and in that way your energy level *can be kept up at all times.*
> *Look like you're glad to be alive.*

Time passed, and while attending a meeting of Nurse Managers, Fran observed the *styles that the leaders used in moving the group toward goal attainment.* She saw *autocratic leaders* . . . leaders who told groups what to do. Groups under this type of leadership were highly productive at times, but they suffered in morale. The *democratic leader* encouraged group decision making. Things did get done, but the process took too long at times. The *laissez faire leader* just sat and let the group direct the activities. This lack of direction resulted in much time being wasted and often nothing of value being accomplished.

There were times when the styles used by the nurse managers varied. Fran saw *idiocratic leaders* . . . those who tended to relate to their staff as individuals, in a one-to-one manner (Stevens, 1980, p. 193). Other times, when meetings were conducted by Clinical Specialists, she saw *technocratic leaders.* These managers saw their role primarily as a clinical consultant. The *bureaucratic leaders* strictly thought that their role was the enforcing of policies and procedures of the institution (Stevens, 1980, p. 193). Sometimes, this style of leadership created anger and hostility from the group.

Fran saw leadership styles varying—*the same individual would assume a different style depending upon the situation.* At first, this appeared confusing, bu

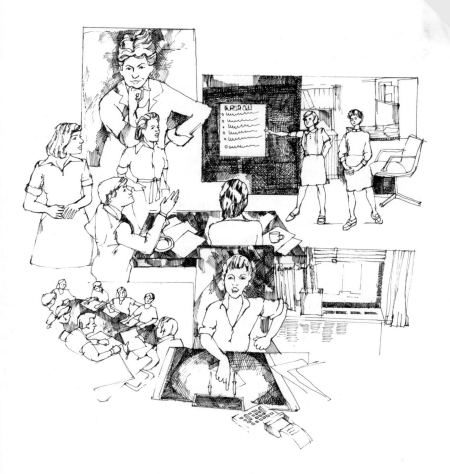

Fran soon realized that those managers using varying styles were the ones who were succeeding. Groups were moving toward *goal attainment*. These leaders had all the positive traits of *looking good, acting good,* but they were able to combine their leadership styles depending upon the situation. These managers did appear to be the most effective.

lity: Self-Worth and
Self-Confidence

After reviewing *leadership behaviors,* Fran felt very overwhelmed. She thought to herself, "How will I ever become such a manager?" From past experience, she recognized that at times she tended to lack self-confidence. In order *to acquire self-confidence* along with most of the other managerial traits, she began to observe individuals who possessed self-confidence. Somehow, this did not seem to help her "find" self-confidence.

One day, very tired and frustrated, she asked herself, *"Who am I?"* This was the first step toward developing self-esteem: *self-awareness.* Rogers contends that individuals who are not "open to their own experience" or are *not self-aware* tend to define themselves *as others see them* (Rogers, as cited in Tappen, 1983, p. 77). Such individuals, who have limited self-awareness, also have limited self-acceptance and *"Waste a lot of time and energy trying to be what they are not,* instead of *recognizing and experiencing all that they are"* (Tappen, 1983, p. 77). To begin increasing her self-awareness, Fran asked herself, "What traits and qualities do I possess, and *what are my strengths and weaknesses?"* As she began to identify these within herself, she also began to obtain additional insight from individuals working with her.

She became *tuned into people's reactions to her behavior.* She actively sought *feedback from others.* This information helped Fran in accurately perceiving herself.

Clinical expertise had been extremely important to Fran as a staff nurse, but she realized that it would take much more than her clinical skills to be an effective nurse manager.

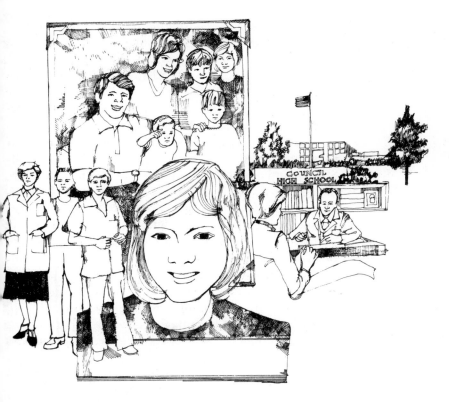

Fran's colleagues were also interested in finding out what management behaviors were important. They decided to observe managers for "successful behaviors." Then, they had a meeting to discuss their findings. Everyone had different opinions as to what "quality behaviors" were important. What they all finally agreed upon was that *each person is unique,* and *each person may function differently under different managers.* Everyone in the group agreed that it was *not* of utmost importance that the nurse manager be their friend, but, more importantly, that she be *unbiased* and *honest.* Fran's colleagues also concluded that a nurse manager should be *intelligent,*

hard-working, and *even-tempered*. They also felt that managers need to be able to *set standards and goals,* but at the same time *be flexible* and *open-minded.*

As time passed, Fran also identified additional qualities that she considered important for a nurse manager to possess. "One must be," she thought, *"self-motivated, persistent, perceptive,* and *diplomatic."*

As her self-awareness slowly increased, Fran found herself able to evaluate her abilities more realistically. She became *more accepting of herself* and *other people* (Tappen, 1983). By increasing her *sensitivity to herself and to others,* she discovered that not only could she identify her strengths and weaknesses, but that her *self-confidence* and *self-esteem* were also improving. This growing self-confidence further helped her to identify her professional and personal goals, and she began tackling them one by one.

So Fran, by examining *who she was* and *who she wished to become,* became more aware of her existing personality behaviors as well as *those that could be further developed.*

Throughout this process of discovering who she was, her *self-confidence* and *self-esteem* evolved.

This, then, was an initial step in becoming an effective, competent Nurse Manager.

Humor

At the first Nursing Management Meeting, after Fran was introduced she was invited to ask questions. Being overwhelmed, she asked, "How do you all keep your sanity in this job, when *everyone* is asking for *everything?* It seems like the verbs of the week are prepare, collect, schedule, answer, process, gather, serve, assume, review, collaborate, participate, identify, attend, listen, and investigate—I don't need to go on."

No one said anything for at least 30 seconds, and then Carol Survivable, Nurse Manager on 3 West for five years, responded with a twinkle in her eye. She said, "Coffee is on me after this meeting, just give me fifteen minutes of your time." As they sat sipping coffee after the Nursing Management Meeting, Carol Survivable said, "Nurses often take things too seriously—remember to laugh at something and at yourself everyday. *Be serious* but not *too serious.*"

"Some things that I and others have used to develop a *good healthy sense of humor* include:

Permitting staff to share jokes if time and place are appropriate

Supplying cartoons

Laughing when something is "funny." If the time and place are not appropriate, find a place and laugh until the *tears flow.*

Touching your colleagues when you laugh—it's both soothing and supporting.

Using *kind or gentle* humor to help others to recognize annoying behavior in themselves."

Carol Survivable related an experience from her past which occurred with a "new" supervisor in the critical care unit. The supervisor had the irritating habit of "rolling up" the monitoring strips that were on the counter and putting paper clips on each one, getting them out of sequence. Since the strips were run hourly and each primary nurse was responsible for documenting arrhythmia changes, everyone complained!

On an unusually busy day, the supervisor offered her help and Carol Survivable responded, smiling, "Yes, could you please unroll my monitering strips and place them in sequence on my clip board? It will save me time when I go to chart." The supervisor laughed and said, "Are you telling me that I've been rolling these monitor strips up for over six months when you *really* didn't want them rolled—that my neatness gave you more work? We need to talk."

By using *kind humor* the whole group was able to open up and discuss other annoying behaviors.

Initiative/Drive/Commitment

At coffee break the next day Fran asked, "How can I get the members of my staff to follow through on something, or . . . really anything? I have nurses who don't get their projects done until two weeks before their Performance Appraisal is due." Another nurse manager from renal medicine laughed and responded, "You're their role model; you have initiative and drive. They need to observe you for another six months or so. Because you are *motivated,* you have a lot of drive; you don't need minute-by-minute or hour-by-hour *instructions.* Trust me, they will watch you and learn . . . or transfer to another unit.

After the manager from renal medicine left for an appointment, Fran sat alone sipping her coffee. She thought, "She is right. I have seldom needed instructions to complete a task once I've been introduced to it. In the past, I asked questions of others or utilized reference material (policy and procedure manuals or medical/surgical texts) when I didn't know or wasn't sure. She's right . . . I don't stand around with my hands in my pockets, and I've never liked 'spoon-feeding.' That's *initiative and drive.*"

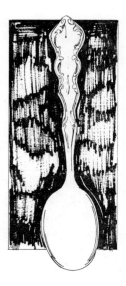

That evening she bought herself a silver spoon to tack onto her bulletin board. Now, whenever she was tempted to "spoon-feed" staff, she would look at her spoon and remind herself . . . "Don't do it. *You are a role model. Staff need to develop the instinct, the power,* and *the ability to follow through* with a plan or task. They need to develop self-motivation without instructions. They need *to drive themselves and not be driven* by you."

"Is initiative and drive all that is needed?" wondered Fran. These traits are important, but they need to be combined with *commitment*.

This became the topic of the next spring retreat. At the meeting, the group was requested to submit ideas for discussion about commitment, and the ideas were written on the blackboard. Discussion went on for over an hour, and when the group finished, the following agreed-upon concepts remained written on the blackboard:

1. *Commitment* is more than just lip service—it requires one to be active at times. It is an internal (or within one's own person) responsibility to *self*, to *nursing*, and to the employing *institution*.
2. *Commitment* does not always mean agreement, but it does mean verbally supporting superiors. Commitment does allow debate, but it also requires upholding the philosophy, mission, and goals of the institution.
3. *Commitment* to self requires a sense of responsibility for the sum total of one's actions.
4. *Commitment* is a choice—your choice.

Assertiveness

"The only way to get things accomplished and to be successful is to be Tough and to Run a Tight Ship!" This seemed to be the motto of Ms. Herrick, the former Head Nurse on 5 West. When the Director of Nursing had told Fran that staff turnover on 5 West was 40 percent, Fran had been surprised; but after working there for six months, she could understand why people left.

Fran could remember when Susan Knew, a new graduate, made a medication error. Upon being informed of the error, Ms. Herrick bellowed, "What do you mean you gave the wrong medication?! What nursing school did you graduate from anyway?" On another occasion when the unit was short-staffed, Ms. Herrick had announced in report, "Since no one cared enough to work overtime this evening, you'll just have

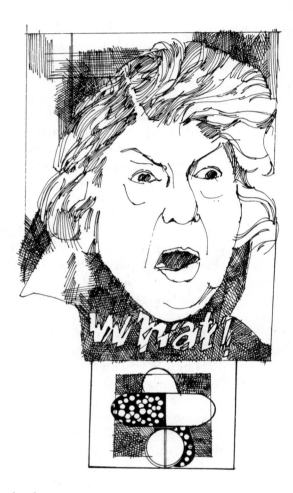

to take heavier assignments. I don't care what you have to do, but you'd better get your work done!" Ms. Herrick's behavior and her responses were almost always *aggressive*.

On the other hand, Wendy Small, the Team Leader on 5 West, was almost always *passive* when interacting with others. On most occasions when the staff asked her questions, her immediate response was, "I don't really know, but I'll ask Ms. Herrick." She tended to avoid direct confrontations, and thus she allowed staff, as well as Ms. Herrick, to dominate her. Although the staff preferred to work with Wendy because she would give her time unstintingly and rarely gave them "a hard time," it had seemed evident to Fran that neither a predominantly Aggressive nor Passive manager was effective in the role. Fran had wondered, "Would a manager with Assertiveness skills be more effective?" She had concluded that before she assumed a management position, she would attend an Assertiveness Training Workshop.

After attending several workshops during her two years on 5 West, and by practicing what she had learned, Fran felt fairly certain that she could be an Assertive Manager. She knew that *Assertiveness* is "open, honest, and direct communication that takes into consideration your own personal rights as well as the rights of others" (Angel and Petronko, 1983, p. 7).

Fran was well aware that although she had learned Assertiveness Techniques, it was not realistic to think that as a nurse manager she would be assertive in all situations. There may indeed be times when she would *choose* to be Passive or Aggressive, depending upon the situation. She knew that it would be her choice and that it would depend upon the decision to be made and what she hoped to accomplish. From the workshops, she had learned that Assertive behavior is not always appropriate and that it should be used with "discretion and good judgment" (Angel and Petronko, 1983, p. 36).

Fran's ability to be Assertive had not gone unnoticed by the Director of Nursing. The Director had observed Fran interacting with other staff and with physicians and had noted how readily she made *eye contact* with others, how astutely she *listened,* and how *clearly* she *voiced* her thoughts. She handled both Positive and Negative feedback without becoming embarassed or defensive, and she could say "no" when that is what she meant. She had learned to *set limits* with her co-workers and staff and could do so without making them defensive. All of these skills enabled Fran to *interact effectively with others* and to *get things accomplished.* As she continued to utilize these Assertiveness skills, individuals interacting with Fran also learned to become more assertive and more effective in their communications.

References

Angel G, Petronko DK: Developing the New Assertive Nurse: Essentials for Advancement. New York, Springer Publishing, 1983

Bass BM (ed): Stogdill's Handbook of Leadership. New York, The Free Press, 1981

Stevens BJ: The Nurse as Executive, 2nd ed. Wakefield, MA, Nursing Resources, 1980

Tappen RM: Nursing Leadership: Concepts and Practice. Philadelphia, FA Davis, 1983

Stage II

What Are the Principles?

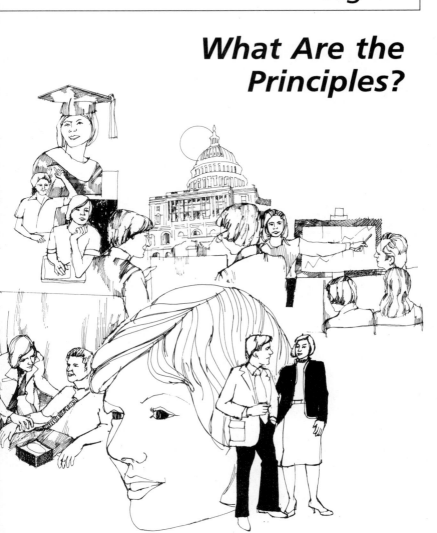

Principles of Champion Development

To *develop champions* effectively, Fran had to know who could accomplish the *task at hand, who was motivated* . . . and . . . *who could be trusted.* Fran always worked very hard *at recognizing situations that needed improvement.* She listened very astutely and often *put into operation worthwhile suggestions made by her people.* When working with people, she made sure her *objectives were clear and to the point.*

Fran knew that any decisions could have a positive and/or negative effect on the accomplishment of goals. Mainly, it depended on *how well staff understood the goal* and whether or not *they believed in the goal.*

Fran believed in *staff creativity.* Her staff never felt like *they were in a box,* but rather they had a real sense that they were her foundation for success. No "we/they" attitude existed. True, there was central direction at the top of the organization, and true, the mission of the hospital was clearly defined, but how these goals were met was up to the people within the organization.

One day Fran was working on her unit, and all of the nursing staff were winding down for the day. Fran made the suggestion that they ought to put all the beds on the floor in a circle. She received quite a reaction from the staff. She heard *why the putting of beds in a circle would not work,* but no one asked her *why it would work.* In a conference, Fran shared with the staff why she had made that comment. She believed that to work successfully with people and to motivate them, one should always approach problems/solutions with a *positive attitude.* Those who always say *why it will not work* instead of saying *why it will work* lack the capability of being effective managers. Fran always encouraged new ideas and provided positive feedback to those who were the *risk takers . . . she gave credit.* She knew that everyone is self-centered and that all individuals are "suckers for praise." Fran knew that her staff wanted to feel good about themselves and that although they needed independence, they also needed direction in their lives. They were creatures of their environment and were sensitive and responsive to external rewards.

Fran quickly learned the ability to *delegate effectively.* This effective nurse manager *confirmed the facts, looked the employee straight in the eye,* and told staff precisely what was expected. She often shared with her employees how she felt about a project. After she let her feelings sink in, she would follow this comment with a compliment on the behavior of the person. She always ended the delegation activity by repeating the goal and establishing a time table. *How this time table*

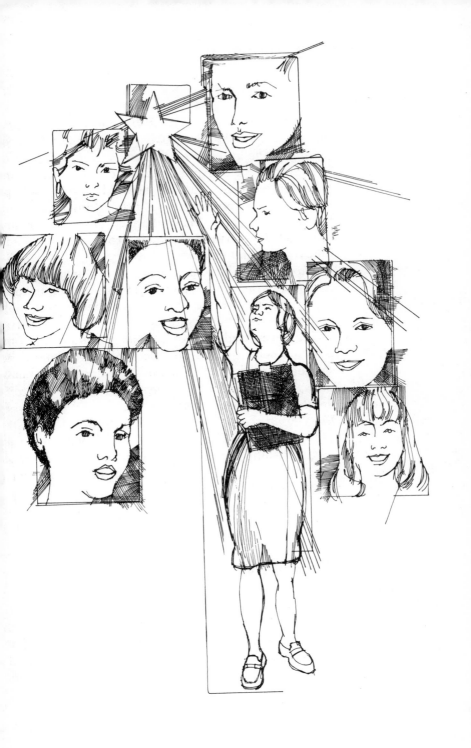

*was to be accomplished was always up to the em-
ployee.*

Fran never put obstacles *in front of people . . . she
put challenges. She set goals and provided for rec-
ognition. She allowed for creativity within her staff.*

Everyone on the unit was treated as a champion.
Fran remembered that Japanese Management kept
telling the workers that those at the frontier know the
business best. Fran knew that a well-run company
relies heavily on individual or group initiatives for
innovations and creative energy.

Planning is valuable, but once it is done, *put it on
the shelf.* Fran was not totally bound by plans. She
used plans as a frame to recognize change as it took
place.

She never made a project *insurmountable . . .* one
that she herself could not accomplish. At times, she
set quotas so that all nurses met the quota. She knew
that all of her staff were *creatures of their environment . . .* They were *sensitive, proud,* and *responsive
to external rewards.*

Fran often rechecked how her staff was doing in
accomplishing the agreed-upon goals. In this process
she always kept her *champions informed on how well
she thought they were doing.*

Principles of Perceptive Communication

Perceptive Communication skills are essential for both
the nurse and the nurse manager. "Communicating
with someone means so much more than simply sending a message and receiving a message; it means *how,*

when, and *what* to communicate," thought Fran. At times it means *reading expressions* as well as hearing the words, for the verbal message may not be exactly what is meant. It means knowing how to *listen* so as to encourage free expression. It means knowing when to be *silent,* for there are times when silence can convey your message better than words. Perceptive Communication means being able to *promote a climate* such that everyone feels free to *exchange openly* their Thoughts and Ideas. It also means knowing how and when to send and receive *feedback* so that both parties can confirm that their message was comprehended.

As a nurse manager, there was little time during the day when Fran wasn't communicating with others—either through words or through her behavior. This meant that she needed to be conscious of what she wanted her messages and behavior to convey. Fran tried to make sure that her messages were *clear, direct,* and *consistent.* Her nonverbal behavior coincided with her verbal messages. She *tailored her words* to the Listener. She Asked her Listeners Questions and she encouraged them to Question Her. This provided her with Feedback and enabled everyone to validate their perceptions.

When communicating a message, Fran was also cognizant of *when* and *where* she expressed herself. There were times when she had to communicate a message as soon as possible. There were other times when the message was delayed because of the moods of the people involved. Fran often thought that she had to rely on her *common sense* to determine when she should communicate. Fran also tried to make sure that *where* she communicated was appropriate for the conversation. If she had to meet formally with someone, she would talk with the person in her office. If the subject or situation was less formal, she might talk

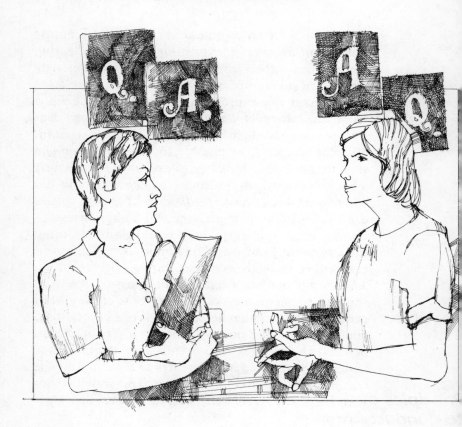

with the person in the cafeteria over a soda or meet in a quiet place on the unit. She tried to find places to communicate where the noise and distractions were minimal. She *ensured privacy* when it was needed.

Fran wanted all individuals to feel comfortable expressing their reactions, ideas, and frustrations. She wanted the staff to be *Active Participants* and to contribute constructively. Because Perceptive Communication is an Interactive Process, Fran knew that in order to facilitate this process and to receive input from others, she needed to be an *Active Listener*. When she spoke with people, she listened with her entire body. She always maintained *eye contact* and she remained attentive. She listened nonevaluatively. She wanted to encourage free expression and to avoid defensive responses. She remained *open* and *interested,* and at times asked questions if she wasn't clear what was being communicated. Her actions made individuals feel that their comments were valuable and were being Heard. Fran *followed-up conversations* by letting individuals know what action or progress occurred as a result of their comments. She frequently did this through memos as well as through verbal messages. She used different methods of communication to ensure that she was heard.

By utilizing Perceptive Communication skills, Fran was able to interact effectively with those around her. Her messages were *clearly heard,* and she received plenty of input from co-workers and staff. This assisted her in her continued growth as a Nurse Manager.

Principles of Group Dynamics and How to Conduct Committee Meetings

There are many types of *Groups* with which Fran became involved. There were *Informal Groups* . . . the nonstructured groups that often met over lunch, at coffee breaks, or during social hours after work. Fran found that she could accomplish a great deal through developing this group *Network.* She listened . . . and *did not talk too much.* When she identified concerns, she *aligned herself with those that were moving in the same direction.*

She associated with the players that she enjoyed and socialized with those who were perceived in the organization as "up and coming." She always worked hard to develop strong *relationships* with successful people. She began to *plan her own informal group meetings,* and over time she realized that people in the organization looked forward to her comments and suggestions.

Fran was also aware that the hospital had *Formal Groups*. These formal meetings had many purposes. Some meetings were conducted just to disseminate information, whereas others were structured to identify problems. Fran had observed that people sometimes assumed different roles in the various meetings, depending upon their perceived status and the purpose of the meeting.

As a Nurse Manager, Fran knew that she *must be prepared to lead*. In her readings, she found that a *Group Leader should bring to any group:*

Warmth and empathy

Attending to others

An understanding of meanings and intents

Acceptance

An ability to link contributions to thought channels (Rogers, 1965, p. 363)

The Director of Nursing asked Fran to chair a Nursing Committee to address the implementation of a Primary Nursing Care Delivery System. Fran requested that the number of committee members be limited to eight. She knew that if the number of committee members increased, she could have a problem in responding to each member of the group.

Fran knew that *"groups should meet in a quiet, comfortable room, where everyone could sit around a table"* (Rogers, 1965, p. 363). For this reason, she chose her office as the location of the first meeting.

"Those who have substantive power *will always try to arrange matters so that meetings are held in their own power spot"* (Korda, 1975, p. 100).

Fran decided that the committee would *meet every other week,* and the *time* would be *limited to two hours.* If the time extended beyond two hours, she knew that her committee members would lose their productivity. She made sure *that the meeting would take place at the same fixed time and in the same spot.* She made sure that the time of the meeting was *firmly marked on everybody's calendar.*

Fran always took a few minutes and *prepared the physical environment.*

Comfort measures that she provided

1. Good light and heat or air conditioning
2. Comfortable seating
3. Good visual arrangements
4. Adequate space for the writing or reference materials of each participant

Convenience measures that she provided

1. Pencils, pens, name cards, etc.
2. A pitcher of ice water and cups

She minimized interruptions by

1. Informing the telephone operator of who was in the meeting and who could be interrupted and who wished to have messages taken
2. Marking her entry door to signify that the meeting was in progress
3. Always checking out the equipment in advance, since she used an overhead projector

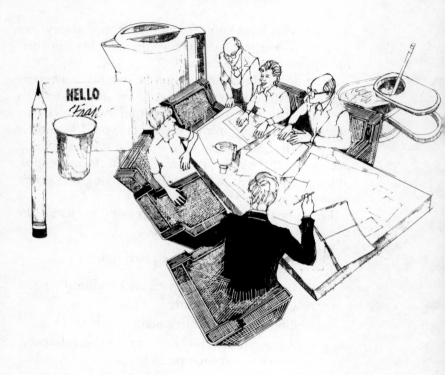

She prepared her agenda well in advance by

1. Distributing the agendas
2. Distributing any documents that needed to be approved or analyzed

She was very aware that when planning an agenda the "star" items would be held until 30 minutes into the meeting . . . . And she always *started business with items that unite* . . . .

Her agenda always indicated the purpose and content of the meeting. Prior to the meeting, Fran and some of the committee members would gather necessary supportive documentation. She also prepared a list of critical questions that could help stimulate the committee's interaction on the agenda topics. She often invited resource persons . . . depending on the agenda topic.

In all situations, the agenda *clearly indicated the purpose and content of the meeting . . . .*

SAMPLE AGENDA

2–4 PM   Place: Fran O'Brien's Office

Members: Jane, Mary, Sally, Anne, John, Peter, Brian, Cathy

Chairman: Fran O'Brien

Invited Guest: Joan Majors, Director of Nursing

1. Review/Revise Job Descriptions for the Primary Nurse.
2. Approve Job Descriptions for the Primary Nurse.
3. Identify Primary Nurses for the pilot unit, based on the job descriptions.
4. Establish time table for discussion with Nurse Managers regarding recommendations for Primary Nurses.

When her committee was first formed, she felt resistance from the members. Nobody really wanted to be on the committee. There seemed to be some time needed for everyone to express their frustrations. In the beginning, Fran allowed the group *time to express their feelings . . . time for the players to get to know one another.* She knew in her heart that the success of any group, *informal* or *formal*, depended on her leadership skills.

Getting Started on the Right Foot

Fran *knew that the leader must set the pace and the mood of the meeting.* She was very clear in stating just what was to be accomplished, using simple behavioral terms. She made statements like, "Each of you has received the Job Description of the Primary Nurse. Over the next 20 minutes, we will review it line by line to see if the competencies are *clear, measurable,* and *attainable.*" She often used an overhead or a chalkboard to help the group focus on the topic at hand.

She became aware that people often sat in the same places at each committee meeting. She observed that if she sat at the head of the table, the next powerful person usually sat to her left. She always made it a point to acknowledge the quieter members of the committee, to elicit their comments, and to stroke them. She was aware that the underlings had to be protected, but she was also aware that Ms. Compulsive Talker had to be controlled. The more assertive staff did not always receive as much positive reinforcement. During the meetings, she consistently worked very hard at attempting to understand what each group member was saying and *feeling* . . . and it was her job to communicate this understanding to the group.

Accomplishing the Objectives of the Committee

Throughout the meetings, Fran maintained a businesslike approach and consistently reduced irrelevant conversation. At times when the conversation strayed, she would stand up, go to the overhead, and underline the topic at hand. Occasionally, she would state, "We're off course . . . and we have only ten minutes left to complete this task."

She knew her leadership responsibilities and saw her function on the committee as:

Focusing the issue

Refocusing the issue when the conversation strayed

Changing the focus when an issue was covered adequately

Recapping the status of each issue . . . the decisions made and the commitments for action

Providing a satisfying windup

She knew that she had to leave everyone feeling great about the progress made. It was her job to bring the group to a closure effectively. At the end of each committee meeting, she would return to the Agenda and summarize the accomplishments.

She ended the meeting always on a *high* . . . with a positive statement such as "We really are great . . . look what we have done. *Thanks for coming;* . . . *without you* progress would not have been made."

Principles of Motivation

The ability to motivate people to achieve goals is key to the successful manager. Before one attempts to motivate people, *one has to be motivated.* Fran began to set objectives. She always knew what she wanted to accomplish each day. She wrote down those objectives. She always tried to look at them *in light of the common purpose and objectives of the institution.* Fran adopted this *goal-setting process:*

Determine priorities.

Identify individuals and resources to achieve goals.

Build relationships.

Seek support, be visible, and let people know of your accomplishments.

Develop an action plan on the determined priorities.

Implement the plan.

Always evaluate and review the outcomes.

The continual planning that she did developed a *bias for action* for her. There were times when she thought she had a great idea but sat on it . . . and let the idea incubate at least 24 hours. By then, her goals usually reprioritized.

There were times when Fran wanted to do one thing, such as attend a meeting instead of meeting her patient care demands, but she cared for the patient instead. This upset her initially, but then she thought, "We do have a central purpose, a central service that we render . . . and to succeed in nursing, we have to *stick to the task* at times. *Organizational conditions need to be arranged in such a manner as to make it possible to achieve organizational objectives, while at the same time orchestrating to fulfill employees' needs.*"

Fran had much to think about. She was a democratic manager, but at times her leadership style varied. She felt that she was a people person, yet at times things just didn't get done. Staff didn't respond, deadlines were not met. She realized that when she became a Taskmaster, things did get done, and on time, but the staff morale usually was low.

McGregor defined these two different types of management. Theory X is "based on the assumption that people are passive and resistant to organizational needs" (Bass, 1981, p. 33). Theory Y is "based on the assumption that people already possess motivation and desire for responsibility" (Bass, 1981, p. 33).

To accomplish goals, management must get things

done through people. The "how" of accomplishing goals is the key to success.

Fran then read *The One Minute Manager*. Although the one minute manager was portrayed as a people-oriented, task-oriented person, he did get things done, and people were motivated. Nurse Managers who were using this approach knew their goals and knew the direction in which they were heading.

Managers using *one minute goal setting* (Blanchard and Johnson, 1982, p. 34) knew what was happening and knew the direction in which they were heading.

1. Agree on your goals.
2. See what good behavior looks like.
3. Write out each of your goals on a single sheet of paper using less than 250 words.
4. Read and re-read each goal, which requires only a minute or so each time you do it.
5. Take a minute every once in a while out of your day to look at your performance.
6. See whether or not your behavior matches your goal.

It all fit . . . *"Look at your goals, look at your performance,* and *see if your behavior matches your goals"* (Blanchard and Johnson, 1982, p. 74).

After much thought, Fran determined her *Role as a Manager*. She would continue participating with people in identifying problems and establishing goals. She believed that people were capable of establishing their own pathways to achieve goals. Goals and directions had to be set, but how these goals were achieved could be at the discretion of the individual. People liked to be praised, so Fran would make an extra effort to recognize achievements, but she would also help people learn from their failures.

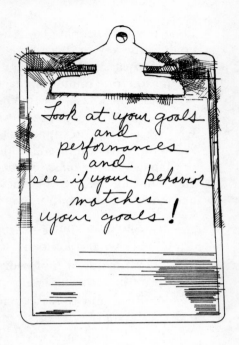

Having attended an evaluation conference in which her boss summarized everything "good and bad" that had happened during the year, Fran decided that people needed to know their errors, *on the spot,* not nine months later. A basic control process was adopted: *establish standards of performance* (meaning: define acceptable work); *measure performance* (meaning: compare the work against the standards); *correct the deviation* (meaning: always, when reprimanding, include a statement about why you are upset).

"Reprimanding is difficult," thought Fran. "I really am uncomfortable telling people when they are wrong. . . ." After some thought, she adopted the following process:

Do it soon.
Be specific.

Tell the person what he or she did wrong and
how you feel about it.
Encourage the person, shake hands, and continue
on . . . . (Blanchard and Johnson, 1982, p. 59)

"People," she thought, "do need praise, but they
also need to know where they stand in the organization on a continuous basis."

She developed a relationship with Susan Strong, a
Registered Nurse who worked in the Nursery. One
day, Susan did not show up for work. This was most
unusual, and Fran tried to call her to see if anything
was wrong. The operator informed her that there was
no phone listed for a Susan Strong. Fran had recognized that Susan was always on time, did all of her
work with gusto, and never carried her home problems to work. Fran decided to stop by Susan's home
to see if she was all right. What she found at Susan's
home startled her. Susan lived in a shack with a small
kerosene heater. There was no refrigerator in the shack.
Susan lived in two small rooms with six small children, who were not all her own children, but yet in
a way they were. She had adopted them, mainly because no one wanted them. Susan was quite ill with
the flu, and the children were attempting to care for
her. "Why didn't you call the hospital and ask for
help?" asked Fran. Susan looked at Fran very proudly
and said, "I know that many of my basic needs are
not met here. Sometimes we barely get enough to eat,
but I never take my home problems to work. . . ."

Fran visited Susan every day, and Susan's health
improved, but Fran also did other things. She quietly
approached the community, and one day a refrigerator was delivered at the door. What Fran was trying
to do was to consider Susan's basic needs . . . and try
to meet them.

When Susan returned to work, she really had a

gleam in her eye . . . the work got done even faster . .
and the quality scores on the unit went up to 95%.

Fran had learned something else about people. They
come to an environment with personal needs, and
these needs have to be satisfied. A manager must un
derstand what is going on with an individual. The
nurse who has struggled all night with a sick infan
may be deprived of sleep, and this nurse may fal
asleep during an educational program on interper
sonal relationship skills just because she was slee
deprived.

Maslow (as cited in Bass, 1981, p. 134) saw the
needs of individuals being satisfied along a hierarch
and believed that one need had to be satisfied befor
moving to another level. Nurses often struggle with
trying to meet their own basic physiologic needs, such
basic needs as getting to the bathroom or finding th
time to eat lunch. Their safety and security needs also
are often threatened. Many nurses carry fears with
them while walking to the parking lot late at night
Nurses enjoy, as does everyone, being a part of th
group and feeling loved and feeling a sense of be
longing. Esteem needs are next, which are very im
portant when one relates this need to motivation
Everyone likes to feel "good" about themselves. Th
highest order of needs is that of self-actualization. Fo
people to truly self-actualize, they must have thei
basic needs fulfilled. To achieve that highest level ma
take years, or it may never be achieved. A manage
must be aware of an employee's basic needs, and mus
attempt to satisfy these needs, before attempting to
move to the next higher level.

"Yes," thought Fran, "As a manager, I will no
only *set goals, reward accomplishments,* reprimand
without incrimination, but *I will accept people from
their own point of view.*"

"Where are they today?" I will ask myself. *"What are their physiologic needs* . . . Are they ill? Is their family hungry? Are their *safety needs* in jeopardy . . . ? Do they feel secure? Has the group welcomed them into the social organization (*social needs*)? How do they feel about themselves (*esteem needs*)? Can they self-actualize (*I've arrived*)?"

So, being a Manager means *moving a group toward goal attainment . . . being creative along the way.* The manager's style varies, depending upon the situation. Some people are *task-oriented* and need to be told to complete a function; and some people are *people-oriented;* but, overall, everyone *thrives on praise.*

How people are directed can be accomplished successfully using frequent *goal identification and praise. Reprimands* should occur without *recrimination.*

Knowing *where people are with their own needs* is an important concept for nurse managers.

Fran decided she will *continue anticipating the behavior of those she works with* . . . and she will focus on a specific individual's problems.

There are certain other traits that Fran continued to work on . . . *individual confidence, integrity, inspiration,* and *persistence.*

Principles of Change

It's just human nature to want things to stay the same! . . . "But I've done it this way for ten years; it's always worked; and why should I change now?" . . . *Change always causes confusion and chaos!*

Fran had heard these comments about change during her experience as a staff nurse, but she knew that as a Nurse Manager and Leader she would need to serve as a *change agent.*

Throughout her nursing career, Fran had seen many instances where nurse managers relied on a crisis intervention approach to resolve emerging problems.

Change was expected to occur usually after a "decree" was handed down from the manager to the staff. Often this change was mandated . . . without considering input from the staff. Usually, only the top "echelons" knew what plan, if any, was to be followed. This approach inevitably resulted in no attention being given to long-range solutions. The confusion and chaos that occurred left morale low and frustration levels high.

"Yes," thought Fran, "It's inevitable that *change is needed at times,* but does it always have to be so disruptive? Isn't it possible for *nurse managers to bring about planned change* rather than chaos?"

She read about change and found that *planned change is that process which "deals with alternatives by choice and deliberation and is distinctly different from change by indoctrination, coercion, material growth, and accident"* (Douglass, as cited in Woodhouse, 1982, p. 303).

As a *Change Agent,* Fran knew that at times she might have to assume additional responsibilities. She might even have to assume the role of a *Risk Taker.* This did not mean, however, that she had to tackle things haphazardly.

The Director of Nursing announced that the documentation of nursing care had to be revised in order to comply with Joint Commission on Accreditation of Hospitals (JCAH) standards. As a staff nurse, Fran had thought that the nursing documentation needed some changes. Other staff members had also grumbled about the amount of duplication required, the inconsistencies concerning what was charted, and how their notes were overlooked by the other members of the health-care team. Knowing that the staff on 5 West was already disgruntled, and knowing that she had some definite ideas on how things could be improved, Fran volunteered to devise a plan for change and to pilot it on 5 West.

Fran was well aware of the Change Process and through her readings learned about the different Models that one could use for change. *For this change to be implemented successfully, everyone needed to win.*

For this reason, Fran felt that the *Normative Change Model* would be the most appropriate in this situation. This model acknowledges and deals with *"People's needs, feelings, values, and potential resistance to change"* (Tappen, 1983, p. 305). Although Fran knew that some staff members on 5 West were disgruntled, she was also aware that they might resist changing their present method of documentation.

To counteract those feelings, she planned *to include the staff as active participants* in the *change process.* This meant that they would *have input* throughout this entire change process.

Fran had acquired much of her understanding of the change process from studying *Lewin's Phases of Change.* In Lewin's work, *the change process* is begun by *initially analyzing the forces for and against the change.* The process is divided into *three phases . . . Unfreezing, Changing, and Refreezing* (Lewin, as cited in Tappen, 1983).

In the first phase of *Unfreezing,* Fran would need to get the staff *to perceive the need for change themselves.* Since some of the staff were already grumbling about the current method of charting, she would need to build upon this in such a way that the group, as a whole, felt dissatisfied with the charting, and yet at the same time felt safe enough to be willing to attempt change. If Fran could get this group "unfrozen" and

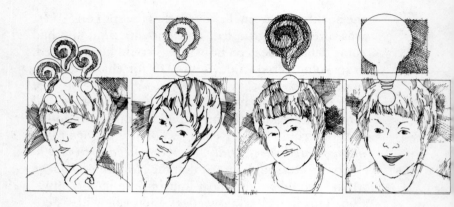

moving toward change, then the planned change could begin being implemented. After this *Changing Phase* the *Refreezing Phase* would *consist of making sure that the change would become a regular part of the routine.*

Although Fran understood these phases, she still was unsure as to what actions she should take—especially during the *Unfreezing Phase.* Fran believed in participatory management, and so she elicited active involvement from the staff in the planning and implementation of this change. By this time Fran was *trusted by her staff . . . unbiased . . . upfront.* Fran knew that this trust would enable her to initiate *group interaction.*

She turned to another *normative change model* derived from Havelock and Lippitt's work (as cited in Tappen, 1983, p. 298) for the needed steps she could use to move the group. These five steps included:

1. Building a relationship
2. Diagnosing the problem
3. Assessing resources

4. Setting goals and selecting strategies
5. Stabilizing, consolidating, and reinforcing the change

Since Fran already had built a relationship with this group, she began by having them verbalize their feelings about charting. As she had expected, there were many who had feelings of frustration regarding the current method, but there were also those who had feelings of fear regarding any possible changes. Fran *encouraged this ventilation.* She answered questions and helped the group to see that a "new" method wouldn't be forced upon them—that, yes, indeed, they could help determine and plan how the charting would change . . . . She was amazed that in the discussion many of the staff's fears were dispelled.

In the group meeting, the staff members were able to begin *diagnosing the problem* (which is the second step of Havelock and Lippitt's work).

After much discussion, the staff compiled a list, which assisted them in *defining the problem.* This list included things such as the following:

1. The nursing documentation frequently did not clearly delineate the patients' nursing problems and how the patients were progressing.
2. An individualized plan of care usually was not documented anywhere—things were passed along verbally at report.
3. Other health-team members, as well as the nurses on the unit, rarely obtained information from the nursing documentation.

After clearly stating the problem, the staff began to *assess the resources* available to assist them. Both Fran and several members of the staff had learned a different way of charting in school and had worked at hospitals that utilized different formats. Fran contacted the Staff Development Department and asked them for help. They were willing to assist. She also met with the physicians and gained their support for changing the charting practices.

It was then time to *set goals and select strategies*. Throughout the entire process, Fran continued to act as a *guide*, as a *resource person*, and as an *energizer* (Tappen, 1983). After listing and discussing many Goals and Alternatives, Fran and the staff finally narrowed it down to one. They made sure that each *goal was clear, specific*, and *measurable*. The group concluded that they would chart their nurses' notes utilizing *nursing diagnoses* and that each patient would have a Care Plan that corresponded with these Diagnoses.

Once the group had decided upon this *goal*, they then had to *determine which strategies* would be used *to implement* this . . . . Again, the group did a lot of *brainstorming*, and eventually they selected optimal strategies to implement this *planned change*.

Fran met with Staff Development, and they helped by developing educational seminars for the staff. These educational seminars were planned to be held on all three shifts over a four-week period, so that everyone could attend. Lists of acceptable Nursing Diagnoses and guidelines to assist the nurses would be made available in several places on the unit.

In addition to planning each step of the implementation, they also decided how and when Evaluations would be conducted. Throughout the *Changing Phase* and *Refreezing Phase*, Fran knew she would need to *provide feedback on their progress*. Since this was being implemented *one step at a time*—first the Nursing Diagnoses, and then the corresponding Care Plans— times were established at the outset for progress reports and meetings. These *meetings* would not only provide the staff *an opportunity to ventilate their feelings* but would also *allow them to know the progress of the change.*

At times it was *necessary to make alterations along the way* . . . but the staff *still continued working toward the original goal.*

Because Fran actively *included the staff, encouraged them to ventilate,* and *openly addressed their fears and concerns,* she was able to *overcome any resistance* and the group was able to *reach a consensus.* By utilizing their *various resources, setting reachable goals,* and *planning their strategy,* the nursing staff was able to implement this charting method. This change *took time* . . . . *It did not happen as quickly as many would have liked.*

But, because it was *implemented gradually and frequently evaluated* along the way, and because *feedback was provided,* by the end of the year it had become the "routine" method of charting. Fran had little question that *Planned Change* could work!

Principles of Power

"Well," thought Fran. "Power is a trait that I must develop to achieve success. What is it and what are the rules that are needed to play the game?"

Bierstedt defined power as "the ability to employ force" (Bierstedt, as cited in Bass, 1981, p. 169). Wrong alluded to the ability to control others (Wrong, as cited in Bass, 1981, p. 169). While driving to work through a traffic jam one day, and surviving, Fran said out loud, "I think that to me, *power means being able to meet and handle the everyday occurrences and demands that challenge an individual* and not to react

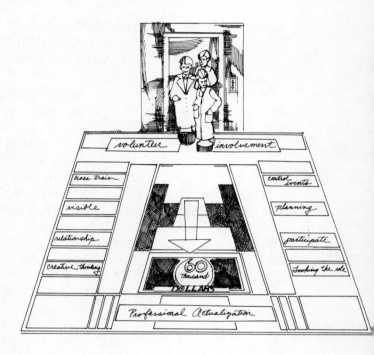

like a paranoid at every imagined threat. Nursing is often disorderly and, at times, chaotic, but even during those times, the powerful nurse manages to live comfortably in the world."

The powerful nurse has a sense of order and plans what she is doing today, and the next day. *The powerful nurse plans.* Insecure people become disorganized in a crisis and often lose power in the process.

It is a game of one-upmanship . . . a game that one can win . . . or one can lose . . . *a game that one can practice daily.*

"How," she thought, "can I master power? Well, . . . it takes practice, and it takes admitting that one wants power. Now, it might be easier to follow the leader, to do nothing, to avoid making ripples . . . but in that situation one cannot lose, but also, one cannot win."

To play the game of power, one should *control events and not the other way around. The environment must be maneuvered.* How can this be accomplished? "Well, I will take the time to analyze my work situation, and especially analyze the players in that environment."

Fran began to notice where the offices were located. It seemed that those most powerful had the offices in the far corners of the building. (Those offices had more windows than most.) After a meeting, she watched who walked off the elevators first. The first individual off was truly the power-holder at the hospital. Fran began to notice that people generally entered elevators by seniority and left it in the order of their relative positions in the power structure. While observing meetings, Fran noted that if she was associated with the leader in the group, instead of with the group, the group generally perceived her as close to the leader. She saw that individuals who sat to the left of the leader were usually powerful, and that those who sat to the right were powerless.

Fran began to gain power. How? She began to actively *participate in the games,* but *she moved the pieces instead of being moved. The environment must be maneuvered.*

Whenever a project or a problem was identified in the committee meetings at the hospital, Fran volunteered. Her thoughts were, *"Getting involved* allows me to assess situations. This helps me expand my name, my worth, and, most important, . . . *it expands my territory."*

When problems were identified at committee meetings, Fran *tried not to look to the past. She always tried to be practical, yet creative.* Dreaming a bit about alternative approaches to problems became her way of setting goals. *The environment must be maneuvered.*

Fran continuously requested new areas of responsibility, and she didn't complain when she was asked to cover other units. "Well," she thought, "I can use these experiences to learn more about the business at hand." Fran was *expanding her territory*.

Gaining power is gaining territory, not necessarily moving up in the organization. Attending meetings, educational seminars, even eating with different people in the cafeteria, provided Fran with *information*. Fran began to learn about the managers . . . who they were and what they really did. She spoke to the elevator operators, always asking: *"What is new?"* Suddenly, Fran knew when the raises were coming, who was requesting what equipment, what games were being played at the upper level. When it was appropriate, she would share some of her tips with her boss. Fran always demonstrated support to her boss, and saw *expanding that relationship* as a vital link to success. At times, her boss asked her to attend meetings with her. During those instances, Fran realized that one can gain power by *associating with a successful person*.

Her boss had gained fifty pounds during her tenure at her job . . . but Fran was determined not to achieve *that* goal. She always looked the role, acted the role. "Please" and "thank you" came easily to her. She worked hard at expanding her bridges, especially the interpersonal bridges. In her committee meetings and on the nursing units, she began to be viewed as a powerful person by her staff.

• • • • •

One day, Fran had an encounter with a resident Dr. Steelshoes.

"Well", said Dr. Steelshoes, with a heavy frown on his face, "I think that it is time for you and me to meet with the attending physician, Dr. Sparks . . . ." "I am right, you know," he said, "and you are wrong. That patient really needed those 10 tests, and I don't care what you say . . . . No nurse is going to tell me how to run my business." Fran didn't respond with anger. She calmly stated that she would contact Dr. Sparks and would set up a meeting with him and the three nurses who were concerned about the great number of tests that the resident ordered per patient. *Coping with crisis in a mature, organized manner results in increased power.*

Fran knew that the resident was going to stack the deck at the meeting, and she resolved to come prepared.

The day of the fateful meeting arrived, and the four nurses left the floor to find Dr. Sparks' office . . . . It was somewhere in the maze of the hospital. They arrived 5 minutes early, and the receptionist, appearing very busy, told them that she would inform Dr. Sparks that they had arrived. Five minutes later, the four nurses were escorted into a large office with windows on either side (a sign of *Power*). Behind the biggest desk one could ever imagine sat a very well dressed man in his 50s. The desk was immaculate. The walls of the office were covered with pictures of fighter planes, planes bombing other planes, and a large plaque citing Dr. Sparks for heroism. On the wall facing the door was a lion's head, mouth opened and eyes foreboding. ("Image and power oriented," Fran thought. . . .) Dr. Sparks sat rigidly in his chair, with the resident *to his left.* (. . . *those that sit to the left of the leader are perceived as being powerful also.*) "They are *stacking the deck,*" Fran thought. Dr. Sparks asked tersely, "And what can we do for you?" Fran noticed the "We," and thought . . . "Can the four of us tackle these two?" Suddenly, she realized that using negotiation process would never work . . . this truly was warfare theory. "I can shoot you . . . . I have enough ammunition, but you will probably kill me."

Controlling Events, Not the Other Way Around, Achieves Power

Fran stood up and said to Dr. Sparks, "I've just received an emergency call and have to postpone this meeting. I will call you back later." Dr. Sparks' shoulders relaxed a bit. The resident, Dr. Steelshoes, continued frowning and just shrugged his shoulders.

Riding down the elevator, the staff nurses asked Fran why she did what she did. Fran shared with them that the outcome of the game that they were playing would have resulted in *one party winning and the other losing.* She said, "We were approaching the event as a *winner-take-all.* We were also *getting even,* and *we wanted revenge!* We really had little concern for the other parties. We had plotted and schemed, and with all the data that we had amassed, and the data that they had amassed, there was no way that there would be a mutual meeting of the minds in that climate."

"We had not viewed the position of the opponent." Fran had not realized this until she went into Dr. Sparks' office.

A few minutes later, Fran phoned Dr. Sparks. She said that she was sorry for interrupting him, and merely asked if he could meet her for a cup of coffee. (*Off his turf and off hers.*) "Well," he said, "I guess so." She had a sense that he was thrown a bit off guard.

"Participating in the game and moving the pieces, instead of being moved, results in power," she thought.

Over coffee, Fran shared with Dr. Sparks her concerns about setting up a warfare situation. She said that she had lined up her guns, and that she had cancelled the meeting because it could have put him in an unfair predicament. She implied that she was concerned. He suddenly relaxed and shared with her some of his concerns, and she shared hers. She asked him what she could do to help him.

Volunteering for duties and expanding your territory and your knowledge at every opportunity achieves power.

The coffee meeting lasted an hour, and during that time, the two talked about Dr. Sparks' problems, including the problem with Dr. Steelshoes, and about Fran's specific nursing problems. They laughed and shared a great deal. They began to look at the problems of too many lab tests creatively . . . and they arrived at a solution, a solution that both could live with.

Creative thinking, looking the role, and acting the role, leads participants to believe that you are powerful.

The coffee meeting ended, and not only did the problem get resolved, but two people established the basis for a friendship. They were able to solve this situation by utilizing *human skills . . . empathy . . .* and *trust.*

That afternoon, the nursing staff and the Department Head discussed the situation. They agreed that *controlling events, and not the other way around, achieves power.*

They discussed a process for negotiations. They all agreed that in a conflict situation they needed to *assess their goals.*

Did they want to win and the other party to lose?

Did they really want to get even?

Or did they want to leave all parties feeling that they had gained.

They agreed that they would generally try to avoid warfare theory. They would set goals, find facts, brainstorm problems, set their position, and always plan their strategy ahead of time. After the tactic was complete, they would evaluate their success.

Fran had learned to use power. She and her staff would always remember the six laws of achieving power.

1. Coping with crisis in a mature, organized manner results in increased power.
2. Controlling events, not the other way around, achieves power.
3. Observing power situations and aligning yourself with powerful leaders achieves power.
4. Participating in the game and moving the pieces, instead of being moved, results in power.
5. Volunteering for duties and expanding your territory and your knowledge at every opportunity achieves power.
6. Creative thinking, looking the role, and acting the role lead participants to believe that you are powerful.

Principles of Risk Taking

"Attempts to lead and success in leading others are greater among those willing to take greater risks" (Bass, 1981, p. 135). "The person who takes risks is one who is closer to achieving than one who maintains the *status quo*," thought Fran. There is truly a spirit of adventure and inventiveness that surrounds the risk taker. It does require energy to invent, *to adventure into the unknown,* but the outcome can lead to new awareness, new products, and future growth for an organization.

Taking risks requires one to act without all of the necessary information at times. When taking risks, Fran tried to amass as much information as possible. She surveyed the environment, looked to the past, and studied her opponents and allies. She attempted to identify all of the alternatives and project possible conclusions. She often asked herself, "If I go this road, where will it end?" She would then think of another path, and do the same thing. She tried to identify the positive and negative outcomes.

Fran sought information, *not only from the top,* but *also from those below her.* She found that the farther down the line she went, the more accurate the information was. She found that those on the firing line usually produced very valuable information.

Whenever she went to change a routine, or even when she went to challenge the organization, Fran always tried to keep her objective in mind, and at times this meant that she had to make adjustments. Some of these risks required moves that were most complex . . . moves that involved the manipulation of people and even situations. As a *risk taker,* she always knew that *she was taking risks* . . . she *knew that pieces on the chess board had to be moved.* She took the outcomes of these changes and seemed to thrive on them.

As Fran participated in risks, she always made sure that her goals were consistent with the organization's needs and values.

She was optimistic and always kept looking for ways around obstacles. She was perceived by her staff

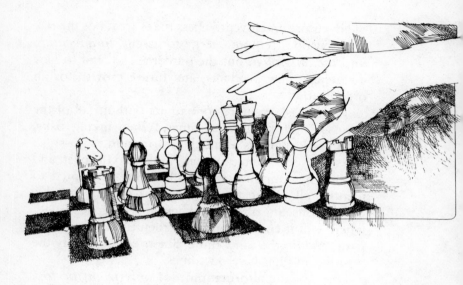

as a self-motivated individual and an individual with self-determination. Fran believed in herself and always believed that she had something of value to offer the organization.

Some perceived Fran as being a nonconformist, but she saw herself as an elastic person . . . a person who took each day as an adventure, and who accepted the challenges of her own personal voyage.

Once risks were taken and decisions made, she accepted the consequences. In all cases, Fran involved her subordinates and tried to give others a sense of understanding as to what was happening.

Fran encouraged her staff to question. She knew that nursing needed role models . . . role models that would not be threatened by questions and not be threatened by the achievements of others working with them. She felt that the *ability to take calculated risks* should be a prerequisite for nursing leadership candidates.

Principles of Stress Management

On Wednesday morning Fran sat looking out her window and thought, "This job isn't what I thought it would be. I'm staying nine to ten hours a day and my work is never completed so I take it home with me. I'm so tired, I don't have time to eat, and yet I've gained seven pounds since I took this job."

When the Director of Nursing, Ms. Major, was making the weekly administrative rounds, she "pulled" Fran aside from the group and said, "Fran, you look tired. Are you feeling OK?" Fran's eyes filled with tears as she responded, "Yes, I just have this headache. I've had it all week. It's nothing." Ms. Major nodded her head knowingly and moved away with the group making rounds.

That afternoon, Diane Smith, the clinical nurse specialist from the Adult Mental Health Unit stopped by Fran's office. "Ms. Major suggested I come and talk to you—that you seemed to be under some stress. She thought maybe I could help you in some way, at least listen, and maybe give you direction. How do you feel about this?"

Tears filled and overflowed from Fran's eyes for about eight to ten minutes before she responded. "I'm sorry, I just can't control my emotions anymore. I usually only cry at home. I'm just under so much stress. I want the staff to have job satisfaction, to perform well, to understand my decisions, and yet continue to develop."

"Fran, I think we have to talk about you and *what you want for yourself.* You've been buffering your staff but not yourself." Fran nodded her head in total agreement and looked at Diane, "You think you can *help* me or is it too late?"

"No way! Can you take the rest of the afternoon

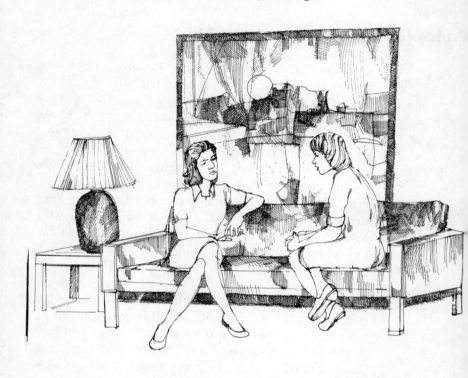

off and come up to my office? You're not going to get work done in this state. We'll look at the progressive stages of stress and take an introspective look at you. You can then decide what you want to do."

That afternoon Fran and Diane covered the stages of stress as described by Alice Dillon (1982, pp. 17–24).

Stages of Stress

Stage 1: *The Honeymoon*—enjoyable stress

Stage 2: *Fuel Shortage*—fatigue and confusion on one side . . . enthusiasm and control on the other . . . "running out of gas"

    a. Job dissatisfaction

    b. Loss of enthusiasm and efficiency

    c. Fatigue

    d. Sleep disturbances

    e. Escape activities (alcohol, smoking, overeating, daydreaming, shopping sprees)

Stage 3: *Chronic Symptoms*—concern about chronic exhaustion . . . develop physical illnesses . . . lose control of emotions . . . "Something is wrong with me."

Stage 4: *Crisis*—symptoms become critical . . . obsession with "your" problems . . . desperate to "get away from it all"

Stage 5: *Hitting the wall*—losing control of your life . . . need help from others

After Diane covered the stages with Fran as outlined by Dillon, they discussed the well-known warning signs of responding to stress: Alarm, Resistance, and Exhaustion.

Diane and Fran talked a long time that afternoon about the healthy responses to stress (Schneider, 1982):

Healthy Response to Stress

1. Know your own body's response—alarm, resistance, and exhaustion.
2. Identify the source of your stress.
3. Change your perception of stress—control the response.
4. Don't let others "dump" on you—be Assertive.
5. Reorganize your job—get some time management training.
6. Add "new" goals for your work.
7. *Don't* demand total satisfaction outside the work area.

8. Develop support networks—group support system.
9. Exercise and relax.
10. Don't brood—move into the future, out of the past.
11. Take mini vacations—to reclaim the inner strengths.
12. Eat a proper diet.

They made plans for Diane to follow-up every Friday for the next month. After one month, they would evaluate the need for their weekly meetings.

After Fran left Diane's office, she went and sat a long time by herself in the quiet of her own office. She needed to get her *own* "act together" if she was ever going to help her staff.

Fran met weekly with Diane for six weeks—she again was feeling good about herself as a person. Fran was ready to move forward. To develop staff to the level she expected them to be and the level they requested, a *stress management* course was needed. She called on Diane to help streamline a program for the unit.

Diane was the leader at the first meeting . . . after discussing possible stressors in each of their lives, she went on to discuss approaches. She said, "To reduce stress one should know oneself and one's stress and should be able to *change* the environment and/or *alter one's behavior.*" The tense group relaxed as one and than another person spoke as to *what* they perceived as the most stressful event in their life. They all followed with their *stressful event* of the *week.* Kind and gentle humor was heard. People listened as others spoke.

Each nurse would develop a plan of action and meet with Fran quarterly to discuss the plan and its progression. Diane would be called for referral or assessment if needed.

As Fran left the meeting, two of her nurses approached her. One said, "Thanks for not spoon-feeding us. We had it all figured out—you were to tell us to get eight hours of sleep and three meals a day, and we would come to work enthusiastic and happy all day long. We'll come up with *great* plans for ourselves."

Fran laughed and replied, "All I ask is that what you do be *measurable* and *realistic.*" As Fran sat down at her desk she thought, "This has got to be one of the better moments in the life of a *Nurse Manager* . . . ."

Principles of Decision Making

Decision making means that the manager makes the *best selection among alternatives.* "The alternatives that we have as managers can come to us from many sources," thought Fran. "The staff . . . the boss . . . our peers . . . our colleagues . . . and definitely the customer—the patient."

In order to obtain input from the various sources, Fran knew she could not attempt the Decision-Making Process in a Vacuum. The *Nurse Manager* must be a *Walking Manager . . . not an Office Manager.* This will enable her to know *who can accomplish the task at hand . . . who is motivated . . .* and *who can be trusted.*

Fran knew that *decisions affect people* within an organization, and that these decisions can have either a *positive* or *negative* effect on the accomplishment of goals. "Major decisions can create major change in an organization," thought Fran. "It is important,

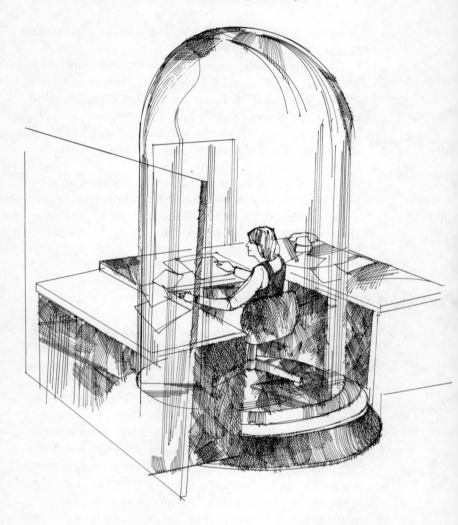

therefore, that decisions be weighed carefully while considering the pros, the cons, and the overall impact on the corporate structure and its employees."

Knowing these things, Fran worked very hard at recognizing situations that needed improvement. She listened very astutely and often *put into operation worthwhile suggestions made by her staff.* When making any decision, she made sure her objectives were clear and to the point. She relied on the following five concepts when making decisions (Newman and Summer, 1964, p. 280):

Saturation

Deliberation

Incubation

Illumination

Accommodation

Saturation. It is not always possible to know all of the facts and alternatives in making a decision, but a competent manager can do her best to become *"saturated"* with all the facts. A *who, what, when, where, why* approach can enlighten the decision-maker and help her arrive at the right decision.

Deliberation. It really is often OK to *stall, weigh,* and *balance* all of the facts and to ask many questions. Deliberation also gives the decision-maker *time . . .* time, perhaps, to gain additional information.

Incubation. Sleeping on a decision, mulling it over, discussing the situation with others, can provide another viewpoint that may alter the original decision. Managers do not have crystal balls, and they cannot forecast the future. Two heads are often better than one.

Illumination. Sometimes an individual will have an idea that is innovative, unique, and appropriate for the situation. A feeling in one's stomach, that old "gut" feeling, should be trusted if that is all one has to draw on in making a decision.

Accommodation. Writing down an idea, rewriting it, sharing it with others, which allows time for thought and discussion, are also helpful.

These concepts assisted Fran in her managerial role and in her interactions with the staff. At one of the Unit Meetings on 5 West, four of the nursing staff requested every fourth weekend off instead of the routine every other weekend off. They stated that, "Each of us has worked full-time for ten to fifteen years on this unit and those years should count for something. We should have more weekends off to be with our families!" The other staff members present (the majority of the unit) nodded their heads in approval, some saying, "That's right!" and "I agree!"

Fran's heart took off at a rate of 114 per minute. "Don't panic," she thought. "Play it *safe; stall* them until you can get all the facts together." She said, "Since all of you are in agreement, let me look at the schedule and see the alternatives. I'll let you know the decision as soon as possible." Fran asked for any other comments, and, since there were none, she dismissed the meeting.

As she left the meeting, she kept thinking of the two objectives she wanted to meet. First, and of the highest priority, was her obligation to the patients to provide quality nursing care and safety. Second was her obligation to staff in providing job satisfaction, and job satisfaction at this time seemed to mean more time off on weekends to spend with families.

That evening, at home, relaxing with a cup of tea, she decided to make a *Decision* using the *Eight Steps for Decision Making* as outlined by Bailey and Hendricks.

These eight steps for Decision Making (Bailey and Hendricks, 1982, pp. 45–47) include:

1. Define the problem.
2. Analyze the situation.

3. Generate alternative ways to achieve your goals.
4. Develop criteria to weigh alternatives.
5. Compare alternatives against these criteria and these goals.
6. Choose the most effective solution.
7. Implement.
8. Evaluate.

With this information, Fran wrote a list of criteria for alternatives. Some of the alternatives, such as hiring replacement help for the weekends and working twelve-hour shifts on weekends, were not possible due to limited resources. Fran also did not have the alternative to close down beds or refuse admissions on weekends.

After weighing all the alternatives with the criteria, she had the solution. She could not give the four staff members off the weekends they requested but she could compromise with a partial solution. At the next unit meeting, after much discussion, the following solution was agreed upon. A seniority list would be hung in the unit . . . when census was low, people could request vacation time, personal time, or time without pay. Implementation would be immediate. The most senior staff member always received the first option. After receiving a "special" granted request, that staff member would be rotated to the bottom of the unit seniority list. At the six-month evaluation there were minimal complaints, and almost everyone seemed content with the "new" system and requested that it remain unchanged.

Although this decision was fairly acceptable to everyone, Fran knew that there are times when decisions have to be made that *result in some of the players on the team losing.* Not all decisions are positive and fun. She could not forget that as a decision-maker she must always *consider alternatives.* She must weigh *who will win* and *who will lose. After researching* as many facts as possible, she must *get on with it . . .* she must not become paralyzed. She must use her creativity and willingness to take risks to assist her in choosing the most optimal alternative. Fran was indeed a *decision-maker.*

Principles of Problem Solving/Conflict Resolution

Fran learned early in the game that *problems* and *conflicts* come with the territory of the Nurse Manager. She wasn't in her new position of Nurse Manager for more than three weeks before open warfare broke out between two of the nurses on 5 West.

From her experience as a staff nurse, Fran knew that the Resolution of such conflicts could either be Constructive or Destructive. She hoped that, by utilizing her perceptive communication skills, not only would this conflict be resolved but the process of *conflict resolution* would lead to increased *creativity,* increased *effectiveness,* and greater *satisfaction* among these two nurses and the rest of the staff.

Before trying to identify the problem, Fran began by examining the individuals involved. Claudia Houston was a staff nurse who had started working on 5 West six months ago. She had come from a large university medical center where she had worked for two years. Claudia was very knowledgeable about all the latest technology, treatments, and medications. Kay Meadows, on the other hand, had worked at a

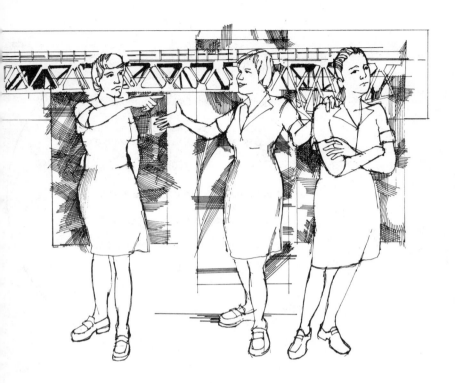

180-bed community hospital in a rural section of Vermont for four years. She had come to 5 West one year ago with a wide variety of experiences.

"With these different backgrounds, no wonder their viewpoints clash at times," thought Fran. "Conflicts often are the result of differences in culture; moral, ethical, and professional values and beliefs; education; experience; and status." As the nurse manager, Fran assumed the responsibility for initiating the process of *conflict resolution*. She utilized the following model.[1]

---

[1]Douglass LM: The Effective Nurse: Leader and Manager, 2nd ed. St Louis, CV Mosby, 1984

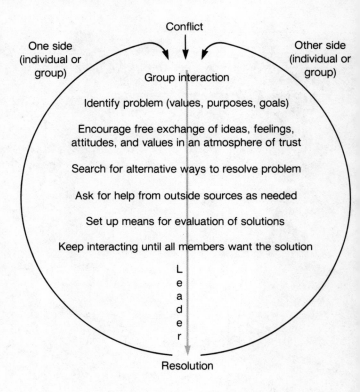

Because both Claudia and Kay were dedicated to their careers and were concerned about providing quality patient care, it was not too difficult for Fran to get them to agree to work together toward resolving their conflict. From the start, Fran made it clear that she wanted a resolution that both nurses could accept. In order to reach this goal, they would need to *communicate their feelings and ideas openly and honestly, respect each other's perspectives (even if they didn't agree),* and *be committed to the process* (Douglass, 1984).

Fran set up some meeting times when the two nurses

would both be working and made sure that another staff member would be able to cover their patients. At the first meeting, Fran helped create an environment where the nurses both felt *safe* enough to state how they felt about each other and what upset them. She attempted to *depersonalize the conflict* by focusing on the activity itself rather than on the individuals involved. It became apparent from their comments that Kay felt Claudia was too rigid and paternalistic with her patients and that she didn't treat them as individuals. Claudia, however, felt Kay was too lackadaisical and didn't provide safe care. After further communication, they were able to become more specific and finally identify the problem. It seemed that when Claudia worked the 11 o'clock to 7 o'clock shift, she often took the same assignment as Kay had on the 3 o'clock to 11 o'clock shift. On two occasions when Claudia made the 12:00 midnight rounds to give medications, she found an elderly patient very confused and trying to find his way to the bathroom. Another time, she had gone into a room to find a patient lying on the floor. Claudia felt very strongly that Kay should be putting waist restraints on the confused elderly patients at night. Kay, however, felt very strongly that patients should not be tied down.

From this exchange, there was little question that this conflict was the result of the different values and perspectives of the two nurses. These values and perspectives were undoubtedly established from past experiences and from feedback the nurses had received. Fran observed, however, that this conflict really revolved around an *ethical issue.*

In this situation, there were basically four fundamental human values at stake. These were (1) *freedom from harm,* (2) *dignity as a person,* (3) *autonomy of self,* and (4) *liberty.* In essence, Claudia felt that Kay wasn't meeting her professional obligation to protect the patient from harm. Likewise, Kay felt that Claudia wasn't meeting her obligations to protect the patient's autonomy and to preserve the patient's dignity. Since every patient is unique and must be treated as an individual, Fran pointed out that an "all or nothing" solution to restraining patients would not be appropriate.

After brainstorming and proposing a number of different solutions, Kay and Claudia were able to agree on what they concluded would be the *most optimal solution.* They both agreed that more extensive patient assessments should be performed by themselves and by their peers. If a patient, particularly an elderly patient, was alert and oriented and had not demonstrated previous symptoms of confusion, she or he would not be restrained. If, however, as it got later in the evening, a patient began to become confused and disoriented, then she or he would be restrained to prevent him from getting out of bed and possibly falling. Kay and Claudia agreed to present these ideas at a staff meeting. Fran suggested that after their presentation, she would ask for three or four volunteers to work with Kay and Claudia in developing a written procedure for assessing patients and guidelines for restraining them. Once this was agreed upon by the 5 West staff, it would then be implemented and evaluated after six months.

By *establishing an environment of trust, encouraging open and honest communication, treating different points of view with respect,* and *attempting to depersonalize conflict by focusing on the activity itself,* Fran was able to assist Kay and Claudia in looking more closely at why they clashed so they could identify the problem and reach an agreeable solution. Kay and

Claudia were then able to include others in their process, which eventually resulted in 5 West being one of the most creative and effective units in the hospital.

Principles of Time Management

For the now seasoned "new" nurse manager, hours turned into days, days into weeks, and weeks into months. Time just seemed to *fly*. Fran found herself staying later and later at work. In the initial weeks she had arrived at 7:45 AM and left at 4:30 PM. Gradually, the time spent at work increased. She was now arriving at 7:00 AM, never leaving earlier than 5:30 PM and *most of the time* she left after 6:00 PM.

Ramona Steel, the nurse manager of the Critical Care area, watched the process for about one month. One evening she stopped by Fran's office at 4:30 and said, "It's time to go home." Fran replied, "I can't. I have two evaluations to do for tomorrow, our Fearless Leader's report is due tomorrow, policy and procedure committee meeting is tomorrow, plus all the little things that came up unexpected today. I need to work at least two more hours." Ramona smiled and said, "What you really need is *my Crash Course on Time Management.*"

Fran: Sure, Sure! From my window, I can see you leaving most every day. You seldom leave late.

Ramona: If I'm leaving too late—it must be a *true crisis*. Tell me—What evening next week do you have free?

Fran: Tuesday . . . I think. Why?

Ramona: Are you sure? I'll need the whole evening.

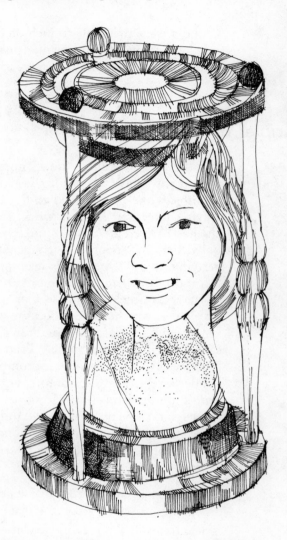

Fran: I'll make it work into my schedule.

Ramona: Good, because you are going to buy me dinner at the Horse & Bridle Restaurant and I'm going to give you my crash course on *Time Management* and you will be amazed how much time you can save.

Fran: Enough to cover the cost of a meal?

Ramona: You can bet the meal on that! I've been in this business of nursing management for seventeen years. I've learned a lot by trial and error. Trust Me! In three days, you'll be looking me up to thank me.

On Tuesday evening Ramona Steel started by pointing at the dinner plate.

Ramona: What do you see?

Fran: A dinner plate?

Ramona: Be more conceptual.

Fran: A circle?

Ramona: Correct, a complete circle. A complete twenty-four hours, or one day. Now what you need to do is put your twenty-four hours in this circle—nothing can be outside. Time is a resource. You need to make time work for you, not against you.

Fran: My days are fairly routine.

Ramona: Good! For one day keep track of everything you do every fifteen minutes while you are awake. Make yourself a sheet like this:

Activity Time Sheet

Time		Minutes
5:30–	Shower	
5:45	Shower	30 min
6:00	Eating	15 min
6:15–	Driving car	
6:30	Driving car	30 min
6:45	Report	
7:00	Report	
7:15	Report	45 min

Fran: It will take me all day.

Ramona: *Sure it will,* but you need to be *conscious* of your time and where it is going if you are going to look at it as a resource. By writing out your time every fifteen minutes you will suddenly become aware of where your time is going. You *need to understand yourself,* maybe you will need a fifteen-minute quiet time with coffee in the morning. Knowing yourself includes your *attitudes,* your *habits,* your *perceptions,* your *values,* your *emotions,* and your *likes* and *dislikes.* I constantly evaluate and analyze my use of time. Whenever I find myself starting to stay later and later at work, I do a *time-activity sheet.*

Fran: I think I'm beginning to think of ways I can save time.

Ramona: Now don't get in a hurry—make a plan. I'll give you the general things I do and you can make your own outline or fit it into your *own* twenty-four-hour circle.

Fran left the restaurant with a package of notes. Upon arriving home, she immediately sat down and prioritized her notes. They went like this:

1. *Make lists.*
   a. A *daily to-do list*—each morning at my desk over a cup of coffee
   b. A *later list*—to be reviewed each Friday afternoon. If it remains important it will be placed in my schedule *to-do.*
2. *Organize folders.* One for each day of the week into which my secretary will place the necessary information I will need for that day. I'll review the folder while writing my *daily to-do list.* (Note: These folders would

include previous meeting minutes for the
meetings scheduled that day.)

3. *Establish schedule.*
   a. *Daily* schedule—will be typed on a card
      by secretary and placed on my desk each
      morning with *folder* close at hand while
      I take fifteen minutes to do my *to-do list.*
   b. *Monthly* schedule—with *target dates* and
      deadlines for those projects or goals that
      can't be done in *one day.*
   c. Allow a *two-hour free time* each day to
      address things that are "true crises" or
      meet with staff about issues that need to
      be addressed.

4. Write out *short-term* and *long-term goals.*

5. Prioritize all tasks according to those *goals.*

6. *Delegate! Delegate! Delegate!* Anything that
   anyone else can do—assist others to learn
   so there can be even more *delegating.*

7. *Avoid distractions.*
   a. Never "work" in the nurses' station—
      too difficult to concentrate.
   b. Put barriers around the conference table
      in the office—to avoid interruptions and
      give privacy during interviews and eval-
      uations.

8. Make *appointments*—make others make
   appointments to see me.

9. *Projects* or *tasks*
   a. *One day*—do them one at a time.
   b. *Longer than one day*—concentrate on one
      project until that portion or phase is
      completed.

10. Recognize *time barriers.*
    a. Answering the telephone—let the unit or patient care secretaries answer, unless they are busy—extremely busy.
    b. Interruptions—*track* them. Are the same people involved?
    c. Incorrect identification of problems—initially take one extra minute to listen carefully.
    d. Socializing—do it outside work except for coffee breaks and lunch. Schedule coffee breaks and lunch with people.
    e. Say *no* if you don't feel qualified or don't have *time to do* added responsibility. Guilt trips are not allowed.
    f. Paper work—try and touch the mail only one time—never more than *twice* except to file it in the waste can.
    g. Staying late—leave after only one hour of overtime, except for a crisis—it can probably be done tomorrow or isn't that important.

Fran gathered up her lists, put them in a folder to take to work in the morning, picked up a book she had been meaning to read for six months, and curled up in the chair with Melinda, her cat.

Time was a resource. It was *her time* . . . she could use it wisely or she could waste it. No matter what she did with it, there were sixty minutes in one hour and twenty-four hours in one day.

Mentorship

Every three or four months, all the nurse managers would get together at one of their homes or apartments for a "thrill and gripe" session. They would discuss everything from problem solving, goals, and objectives, to food and clothing styles. *Internally,* Fran felt good after these times and always went home feeling like she was part of a team.

At one of these meetings, the subject of mentorship came up quite accidentally. As the group discussed role models and "ideal" leaders, it suddenly occurred to Fran, "We are no longer simply discussing role models . . . we're discussing mentors—'that special someone who guides, advises, and promotes our careers'" (Vance, 1982, p. 10).

The group surprisingly discovered that seven of the nine nurse managers present had mentors; however, very few were mentors themselves. "Maybe the reason we have the self-esteem, security, and confidence to be where we are in our careers is because someone took the time and energy to mentor us," Margaret suggested. Sara added thoughtfully, "Early in my career, I considered my mentor very important. She was that person I could always call and depend upon for an objective response and perspective."

"My mentor was excellent at providing *feedback* and *inspiration,*" John agreed. "She helped me to feel excited about myself. She was older; I think she saw me as the future, and she was investing something in that future."

"I don't think of a mentor as being someone older," Lee admitted. "I picked my mentor in school. She was actually about my age, but she was an educator and was much more *scholarly advanced.*"

Fran asked, "Don't mentors pick their own protégés? I felt mine selected me. It was a mutual, non-verbal agreement that just occurred. Now, it is my *professional responsibility* to *support* and *strengthen* someone else."

"Maybe, but the *time* and *energy* needed to mentor

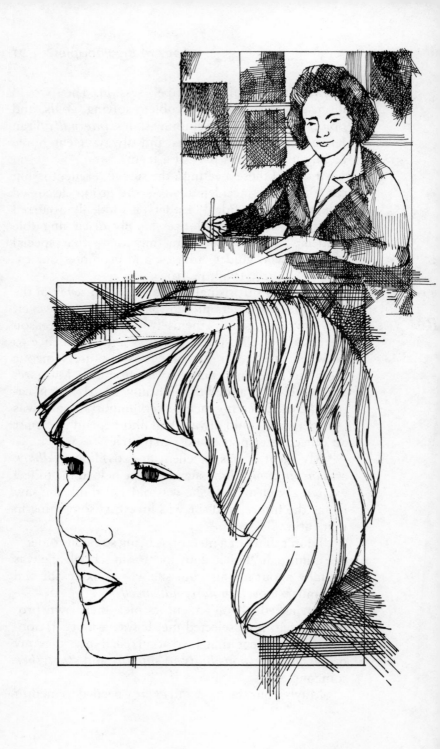

someone seems like *hard work*. When I leave the floor and go home, all I want to do is relax," Sara insisted.

As Fran drove home, she thought about all that had been said and then reached a personal decision. To date, all she had done was take from the system. "I have experience, Yes, I am willing to *support* and *guide* someone. I have the energy. I feel *mentoring is important*—I will schedule the time," she thought. "I will try to be more sensitive to the needs of others and this may even help push others into being mentors."

References

Bailey JT, Hendricks DE: Decisions, decisions: Guidelines for making them more easily. Nursing Life 2(4):45–47, 1982

Bass BM (ed): Stogdill's Handbook of Leadership. New York, The Free Press, 1981

Blanchard K, Johnson S: The One Minute Manager. New York, William Morrow & Co, 1982

Dillon A: Reducing your stress. Nursing Life 3(3):17–24, 1982

Douglass LM: The Effective Nurse: Leader and Manager, 2nd ed. St Louis, CV Mosby, 1984

Korda M: Power, How to Get It, How to Use It. New York, Random House, 1975

Newman WH, Summer CE: The Process of Management. Englewood Cliffs, NJ, Prentice-Hall, 1964

Rogers C: Client Centered Therapy. Boston, Houghton Mifflin, 1965

Schneider S: Curing burnout while you work. Nursing Life 2(5):38–43, 1982

Tappen RM: Nursing Leadership: Concepts and Practice. Philadelphia, FA Davis, 1983

Vance CN: The mentor connection. The Journal of Nursing Administration 12(4):7–13, 1982

Woodhouse DK: Change. In Marriner A (ed): Contemporary Nursing Management: Issues and Practice, pp. 302–307. St Louis, CV Mosby, 1982

How Do I Play the Game?

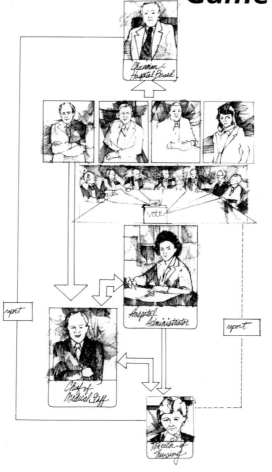

Organizational Dynamics

Fran felt like she was finally getting "into" her job. In just four days, her Management Orientation would be completed. Today she was meeting with Tara Lawton, Coordinator of Staff Development for Nursing, to discuss and evaluate the whole nursing management orientation.

They met in an empty classroom and their conversation went like this:

Tara: How is it going for you?

Fran: OK . . . I guess. Little things keep coming up that I didn't expect or hadn't been told about. I kept the list for you.

Tara: Good! Were you able to wade through the *Hospital* policy and procedure books?

Fran: Believe it or not, I got through that big blue book last week.

Tara: Did you say *blue* book?

Fran: Yes, blue with white lettering.

Tara: Now wait—*Nursing* Policy and Procedure manual is *blue* with white lettering; the *Hospital* Policy and Procedure Manual is *white* with blue lettering.

Fran: I was supposed to read the *Hospital* Policy and Procedure Manual? You're kidding, of course!

Tara: No, I'm not! Being a Nurse Manager you need to know more than just Nursing Policy and Procedure. You are *accountable* and responsible for knowing *Hospital* Policy and Procedures. I know it may all seem very *boring* and *heavy, but* it is *important* that you know the inner workings of the hospital.

Fran: You *are* serious.

Tara: You can bet your next paycheck on my seriousness. . . . I apologize, I probably didn't make it clear that I wanted you to read both the *Hospital* and the *Nursing Policy* and *Procedure Manuals.*

Fran: I'm so sorry!

Tara: Please—don't get upset. We are scheduled to be together all day. I wasn't sure what we were going to do with all that time. Right now we'll review the *pros* and *cons* of the Nursing Management Orientation—that should take us about one and a half to two hours. After that, we'll take a short break, then come back, open up these *white* and *blue* manuals, and go over some of the "heavy" material like *Organizational Dynamics.*

Fran: Are you sure?

Tara: Listen, I could use the review. It's great to know the answers when people ask me questions in orientation about trustees, hospital president, philosophy, mission, and anything else that crosses their minds.

Two hours later both Tara and Fran could be found at the table with the *Manuals* in front of them taking notes.

Fran: This is not the sort of thing that can be memorized, but I do remember a lot of this from school. Somehow, it is beginning to make sense now that I can apply it to *this hospital.*

Tara: Let's see what the manuals say about:

The Role of Trustees in Relation to the Mission of the Hospital

The Board of Trustees is fully responsible, legally and morally, for the institution and for the services that are provided. They are responsible for:

1. Determining the overall goals and long-range plans of the institution
2. Determining the major policies of the hospital in relationship to the health needs of the community
3. Maintaining proper professional standards in the hospital and monitoring these functions through a quality-assurance program (This is a system that monitors the effectiveness [or quality] of the care given to patients.)
4. Assuming general responsibility for adequate patient care throughout the institution

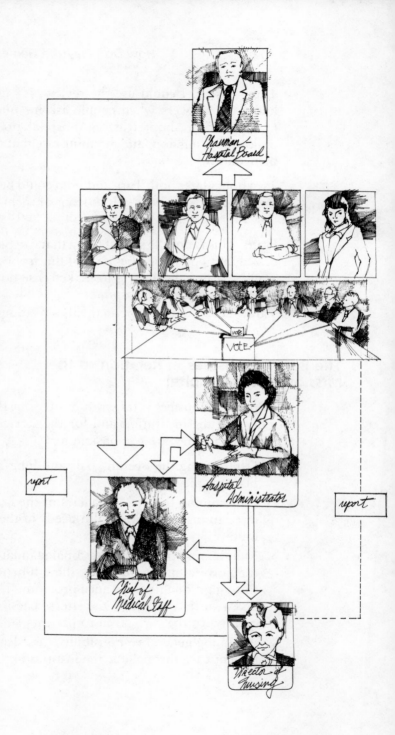

Chairman –
Hospital Board

Hospital
Administrator

report

report

Chief of
Medical Staff

Director of
Nursing

VOTE

5. Providing adequate financing of patient care, maintaining financial stability, and assuming business-like control of expenditures (Rowland and Rowland, 1984 p. 723)

The vital role of this governing board is to operate the hospital *in such a manner that satisfactory patient care can be rendered.* It is the responsibility of this Board to maintain a Quality Medical Staff and to maintain standards that will be met through the employees of this institution.

Fran: I see the Board of Trustees' philosophy also includes a commitment to the medical educational program, nursing educational program, and medical research. That's great!

Tara: The Board of Trustees meets monthly. They have developed functioning committees, some of which are:

Financial Planning
Public Relations
Quality Assurance
Long-Range Planning
Board/Medical Staff Committee

You'll learn, Fran, that sometimes we'll have a project planned and all of a sudden we hear it is "tied up" in Financial Planning. Well, this is that committee, and trust me, they are powerful. Our Director of Nursing participates on the Board of Trustees, and she has contributed greatly in the decision-making processes of the institution. During planning and review of goals, she often solicits the opinions of those of us in nursing management.

Fran: So, . . . all the more reason for me to know how the system works.

Tara: Moving on to:

The Role of the President/Hospital Administrator

Tara: The President/Hospital Administrator is selected by the Board of Trustees. There are basic minimum standards defined by the hospital licensing statute that define the educational qualifications of the Administrator. As you can see, the manual just says, "there are basic minimum requirements." This administrator came with a Master's Degree in Hospital Administration and eleven years of executive experience.

Just for your inside knowledge. He believes in being *visible*—so you can expect to see him on your unit at unusual times. They say he stops by the hospital for ten to fifteen minutes every weekend.

Fran: From my past experience, I know the physicians are important because they admit patients to the hospital and because they provide services such as surgery, echocardiograms, and so on, which bring *money* into the hospital.

Tara: Let's discuss:

The Role of the Medical Staff

Tara: In most hospitals there is an elected individual called the *Chief of Staff*. This is usually a *tenured* physician, who is by virtue of his position responsible for the *management* of the medical staff. This individual usually participates as a member of the hospital's Board of Trustees. Our hospital is no different, our Chief of Staff is on the Board of Trustees.

There is a committee that delineates privileges for physicians. An Active Medical Staff Member has full hospital privileges, is responsible for some administrative activities, can vote at the medical staff meeting, and can also hold office. This physician is *expected* to serve on medical staff and hospital committees.

An Associate Medical Staff Member is usually a new physician who is practicing at the hospital. He may *not* hold office, and he is usually expected to serve on committees. This is the norm; the exceptions you'll probably hear about by rumor and gossip.

The Courtesy Medical Staff consists of physicians who are active elsewhere and have the privilege of admitting patients only on occasion. They usually have no administrative functions within the hospital.

The Consulting Medical Staff Members are those physicians who can admit patients and who are recognized for their unique professional expertise. These physicians are usually based at one of the large medical centers in the area, and they are willing to act as consultants to other physicians.

The House Staff consists of interns and residents. These physicians (if they pass their medical boards) are salaried by the hospital and are supervised by the attending physicians. They elect or appoint a Chief Resident, who intercedes on behalf of the residents should the need arise. A word to the wise:

only go to the Chief Resident after you have *firs* attempted to resolve your problem with the indi vidual House Staff physician.

Fran: Now to:

The Role of the Director of Nursing

Tara: The Director of Nursing, Joan Majors, wa: chosen by the President/Administrator with inpu from a Search Committee. The members of the searcl committee were nurses and physicians. Our Direc tor of Nursing reports directly to the Presi dent/Administrator. She does not report to the Chie: of Staff, but there is no doubt that strong informa linkages exist with the Chief and the physicians.

Although our Director of Nursing was hired by the President/Hospital Administrator, you will finc in certain Corporate Models that the Director o! Nursing reports directly to the Board of Trustees and has the ultimate responsibility for the man agement of her department. Usually in these situ ations, the nursing directors that are chosen rep resent many years of educational and practice experience.

Fran: Let me describe my:

Role as the Nurse Manager and My Involvement with Others

Fran: I need to know not only the key physicians, but I also need to work hard at developing credi bility with them. Nurses today are not handmai dens, but are competent, astute practitioners. To increase my credibility, I need to inform physicians of significant clinical problems in a timely manner. I need to inform my supervisior of significant events, so that she may carry this information upward to the Director of Nursing, who has the ultimate accountability for the Department. The Director of Nursing needs to know significant events because she has the full management responsibility for the operation of her department. The Director of Nursing is ultimately accountable to the President /Administrator of the institution.

Tara: You've got it . . . in a nutshell, that's it!

Now that we are on a roll, let's move onto *Philosophy, Purpose,* and *Objectives.* When Joan Majors, the Director of Nursing, came here she immediately formed a committee, which she chaired, to develop a philosophy of nursing. I volunteered to be on that committee . . . To Participate.

At the first meeting, Ms. Majors told us, the committee members, that the *"Philosophy of Nursing Must Emanate from the Philosophy and Mission of the Overall Institution."* The statement that was developed included the Values and Beliefs that influenced the practice of nursing in this hospital (Stevens, 1980, p. 23). The information developed became the Framework for Nursing Practice. There are many elements that we included in the development of this Philosophy of Nursing:

Beliefs about nursing and nursing practice

Administrative theory

Organization and model of nursing care

Beliefs about the right of patients and personnel

Educational needs of patients, family/significant others, personnel, students

Appropriate use of the environment and human resources

Spiritual Needs of Patient

Ethical Considerations in the delivery of nursin
care

Interdisciplinary relationships (National Leagu
for Nursing, 1980, p. 1).

We worked hard on the Committee to develo
a *Philosophy of Nursing* . . . and what we agree
upon was:

A Philosophy of Nursing

Tara: The mission of the hospital is "to provid
optimum patient care services." The Departmen
of Nursing adopts this personal-centered philoso
phy.

This philosophy is based on the belief that a
persons—patients and health-care providers—de
serve to benefit from an individualized, holistic ap
proach where the resources of each person are uti
lized to the maximum. The whole person (spiritua
emotional, physical, social) is considered.

We support a participatory climate where nurs
ing is respected as an independent profession. Nurs
ing has a specialized body of knowledge that i
operationalized by the nursing process. Nursing act
in a collaborative manner with all other Profes
sionals, Disciplines, and Departments.

Through a decentralized process, the nursing de
partment will assess, plan, implement, and evaluat
its professional practice under the direction of it
nurse administrators, nurse researchers, nurse prac
titioners, and nurse educators.

We assess our professional practice via commit
tees in which nursing administrators, nurse re

searchers, nurse practitioners, and nurse educators develop a scientific basis for all nursing decisions. Enlightened decision-making enhances our responsibility to act as patient advocates.

We plan nursing practice via nursing administrators who:

Determine nursing's response to the needs of the community

Respect the rights of each individual nurse

Provide a framework for practice, including department structure, mode of care delivery, staffing, and support of the recommendations of the Professional Organization

We implement nursing care via the primary nurses who practice professional nursing. Autonomous registered nurses use the nursing process to deliver effective patient care, with respect for each patient and family.

We evaluate nursing care in terms of patient outcomes. Nurse researchers and nurse educators foster a climate where all levels of nursing personnel assume responsibility for their own professional growth and development. Professionally developed practitioners alter their interventions appropriately, facilitating successful outcomes.

Necessary resources with the Department of Nursing participate with the Primary Nurses to provide for cost-effective quality nursing care.

We believe that each nurse and each patient offers a unique contribution of personality, talents, values, and goals. We assume the responsibility of working together to build, from these gifts, an environment in which the mission of "optimum patient care" can be fulfilled (Warner, 1983).

The Statement of Purpose and Objectives for Departments of Nursing

Tara: Those of us on that committee believed strongly that the philosophy of nursing was necessary before goals and objectives of nursing or of the units could be addressed.

Fran: You're saying that the purpose flows from the *Philosophy of Nursing?*

Tara: *The purpose of the Department of Nursing is to provide quality nursing care services for all our patients.* Objectives flow from the purpose . . . from the overall purpose of the Department of Nursing. There are *General Objectives* . . . pertaining to the entire division, . . . and there are *Specific Objectives,* pertaining to a particular nursing care unit. Fran, the critical aspect of writing objectives is *that objectives be observable, measurable, and realistic. . . . "A behavioral objective expresses the intended outcome of an experience"* (Reilly, 1980, p. 33).

What is most important is that the stated objectives, whether they are permanent (forever) or temporary (to be accomplished within a year), need to be *measurable.*

It is up to the Director of Nursing, with Management staff input, to develop a way for all of the departments' objectives and the units' objectives to mesh. . . . Objectives built upon one another can be specific to either the individual needs of the patients or the personnel served by the department or the specific nursing unit.

Fran: So for my unit, I need objectives that are *measurable, observable,* and *realistic.* Some examples that I could develop for my nursing unit would be:

1. To improve quality scores by 10 percent this year
2. To have all staff CPR-certified by November, 1986
3. To obtain 100% compliance with the new Nursing Documentation—utilizing Nursing Diagnoses and Care Plans
4. To begin having staff perform peer evaluations. By the end of the year, everyone should have received and written at least two peer evaluations.

My head is beginning to swim.

Tara: Time to take a break! Let's go to lunch.

Organizational Systems

Tara: Part of the reason why I had set so much time aside for you today was because I felt it was important to cover the organizational systems of this hospital . . . past, present, and possibly future systems. We are currently decentralized and decision making takes place at the lower level. We have been decentralized for eight months and have worked some of the "bugs" out of the system.

Because you'll hear about it, especially when someone isn't sure who to report to, I'll give you the history.

The Director of Nursing, Joan Majors, along with the help of others in nursing management, created an organizational system . . . a *system compatible with the philosophy, framework, and goals of the hospital and nursing department.*

Nurse Managers, because of their involvement from the beginning, understood the entire organization . . . not only the nursing part. They began to understand the interrelationships of other departments . . . . They saw that nursing did not function in a vacuum . . . they saw that nursing had to cope with many dual forces.

The organization that developed defined clear lines of authority and clear lines of communication. It also helped in reducing duplication of efforts . . . . Two people were not doing the same job at the same time.

All the while, the organization remained *fluid.* As the need arose, changes were made. The focus of the organizational goals was to maintain quality, to improve constantly, and to eliminate problems.

Centralized Systems

Tara: *A Centralized Structure had been the mode of operation for many years . . . .* This type of structure kept the control at the top, but carried with it many problems. Those at the Director and Associate Director level commanded considerable power. Often times, decisions made at the top did not reach the bottom and so many decisions were not accomplished. It looked something like this:

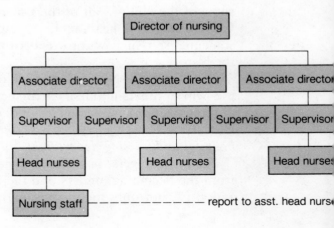

Fran: This is the system I know, and you are correct—most of the decisions are made at the top. I would frequently read minutes to see how long it was until a decision came up at staff meetings . . . three to four months was the norm.

Tara: Change does not come easy, so everyone was anxious for about the first two months, but here is how we got the *Decentralized System* going.

Decentralized Systems

Tara: A committee, organized by our Director of Nursing, adopted a belief that those in nursing had to work as a team in order to foresee and solve problems. The complete aim of all in nursing management was to help the staff do a better job. The Decentralized System placed the authority for decision making more toward the local (staff) level. Money was saved because there were fewer needed in the authority level. The Nurse Manager was expected to manage and to make major decisions. It was hoped that this type of organization, by placing the decision making near the action, would create an environment where people could grow. In just the eight short months since it was implemented, I've seen what I thought was stagnant staff blossom and grow. The chart now looks like this:

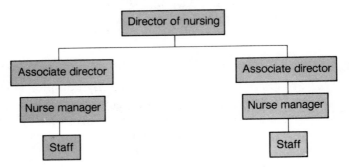

There could have been problems if the Nurse Managers were not prepared in management, but they were. This type of organization provided very limited supervision from those in upper management.

Those in *Line Management* (The Associate Directors' relationship to the Nurse Manager) have direct responsibility and authority for the management of their units. They enforce agency policies and guide and evaluate their subordinates.

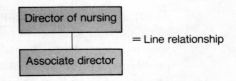

Those in *Staff Positions provide support* to those in line positions. They function very much as consultants . . . they can advise, encourage . . . but do not hold the total authority for decisions that affect the agency.

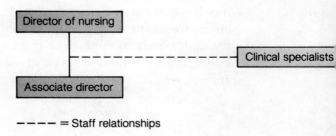

Matrix Systems

Tara: In some highly complex organizations, matrix reporting relationships exist. *Matrix . . .* implies reporting to more than one individual. This type of reporting relationship at times can cause confusion on the part of the subordinate. Why? It really can be difficult reporting to two bosses. In reality the Matrix Organization has occurred for many years.

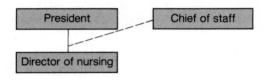

In this hospital, the Director of Nursing has had a direct reporting relationship with the president, but has had an indirect relationship (maintains communications, advises, etc.) with the Chief of Staff.

This situation is not obvious on the organizational charts, but an informal relationship between the Director of Nursing and the Chief of Staff actually does exist.

Matrix reporting relationships work very effectively at the high levels in this organization, but most of our problems are occurring at the lower level.

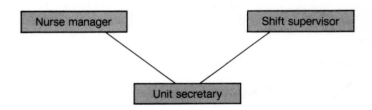

It can be difficult for the unit and patient care secretary to report to two bosses . . . . In this situation, there is an overlapping of communication, direction, and goal setting, making it very frustrating for the unit and patient care secretary on the job.

The organizational chart has been developed. It is a decentralized system that encourages decision making at the lower level. *It is available and visible* for all of the employees in the institution. So are the philosophy, purposes, and objectives of the hospital, nursing department, and each unit.

The Chart has been very helpful as problems have arisen. It has identified those who are available to advise, consult, or cooperate.

Fran: Every organization has *Informal Chains of Command.* I know individuals exist who are not visible on a chart, but who really wield the power within the institution. From my experience, *the Informal Structure* has been the actual working structure at times, when it came to the decision making. I learned from the past, it is important for me or anyone aspiring to be a manager, . . . to take the time to identify *who is part of that Informal Network.* . . .

Tara: You're off to a good *Start* by identifying that informal network. Can I help you in any way?

Fran: You sure can! Tell me who has been here the longest. Who has survived all the changes?

Developing Standards of Care (Quality Assurance)*

Fran, as a new nurse manager, raised many questions about *Standards of Care* at the first Nursing Council Meeting. When she questioned her peers, the group

*Contributions from Nancy Voss-Coleman

responded in almost total unison, "A day with Jane Quest is just what you need. She'll answer your questions."

Jane Quest sighed with relief as she talked to Fran. It had been nine months since she, as the Assistant Director of Nursing, initiated the *Quality Assurance Program.* Today, she received positive feedback from the staff: the nursing audit on 4 East demonstrated 89 percent compliance for the month of March. This fact became more meaningful as Fran examined how Jane strived for quality in the nursing department.

Quality assurance was not new to Jane. She had been in nursing for fifteen years, the last six in administration. Jane learned years ago *that nurses need to be accountable for their work.* She knew that *Quality Assurance is an evaluation of services provided and the results of such services compared to accepted standards* (Urdang, 1983, p. 917). Nine months ago, Jane started introducing ways by which her staff could provide such quality in their patient care. She realized that optimal quality care would vary in each nursing unit in the hospital. She further realized that each hospital in the area and in the nation would have different standards to measure quality. Jane's theory was that no one individual program would ensure quality, but a combination of systems and programs could be most effective in meeting such quality needs. She instituted the following mechanisms based on the results of a nursing staff questionnaire:

Nursing audits
Nursing rounds
Patient questionnaires
Professional role expansion

Nursing audits are used to inspect the actual tasks of nursing care rendered and to compare them to the

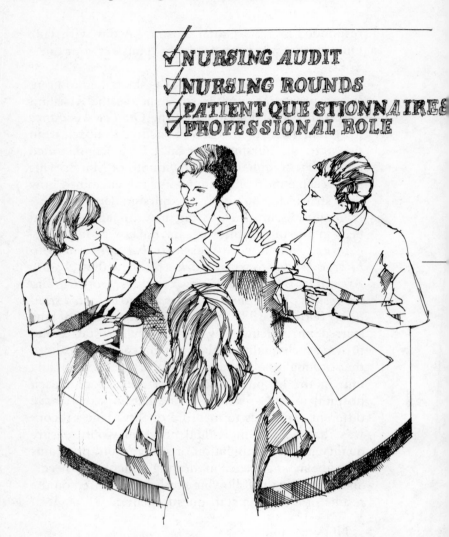

standards and criteria already set by JCAH, ANA
and NLN. With the results of the comparison, Jar
could see where compliance was obtained and when
deficits existed. Not only could she see it, but the sta
would be able to observe it as well. This audit the
enabled the staff to provide compliance for the defici

noted, and the end result would be better nursing care and, ultimately, quality nursing care.

On 4 East, the staff was asked to "brainstorm" and create lists of all those tasks and nursing functions done during their shifts. Jane met weekly with this staff to first break down the list into similar categories and then to organize the tasks into a workable audit sheet. Checkmarks would be placed next to each item indicating "yes, the task was completed," "no, the task was not completed" or "not applicable." Jane used JCAH and ANA standards as guidelines for formulating the tasks into an audit sheet; therefore, compliance to JCAH was established at the staff level.

The staff's first audit showed a 46 percent compliance, and Jane's hardest work began: *motivating the staff to increase compliance.* She needed to reinforce that current work was good, but staff needed to initiate ways to improve the nursing care that was provided. She felt that telling the staff to comply in this or that category would probably not lead to improvements in quality care. The staff met almost daily to see where they could make improvements. As their audit results approached 100 percent compliance, more positive feelings of accomplishment were shared with Jane. Jane did not let this opportunity for reinforcement slip by her: *she publicized these improvements at executive meetings* and *in the hospital newspaper, and rewarded the staff with a free luncheon.*

The second mechanism Jane developed was *Nursing Rounds.* On 4 East, nursing rounds were integrated with the nursing audit. Jane selected nursing rounds in order to highlight the positive effects they could have on quality care. Jane met with the staff and then defined rounds by the following criteria:

1. The team report between primary nurses will be 25 minutes and will occur while walking

from room to room. Charts will accompany the change of shift primary nurses.

2. Teaching Rounds will occur at least once a day and will consist of discussing specific problems that are present in the care of current patients.

3. Nursing Rounds will be held every other month and consist of a lecture concerning current clinical issues. All nursing personnel will be invited.

Utilizing the above criteria, the staff on 4 East wa able to solve some of their most frequently state problems. Brief inspections of each patient as the sta walked from room to room eliminated those state ments that used to occur at the conference room re port: "I don't remember how much fluid is in M Smith's IV bottle"; "I told the aide to empty Mr Renshaw's Foley bag and record it" (which the sta found later was not done); and "The abdominal dres ing on Joe Porter is dry and intact" (when it wa saturated with blood one hour post report). The of going shift felt obligated to finish all responsible task because they knew the patient would be directly ol served at change of shift. The on-coming shift ex pressed less negative comments about the previou shift's unfinished work because they could see it wa done.

The Teaching Rounds served the purpose of solvir problems where each nurse felt alone in taking ca of "her" patients. Rounds provided an arena whei a free exchange of concrete ideas helped increase tl quality of care given to each patient. They were hel informally, often over coffee breaks, and usually tl knowledge exchanged was put into practice the san day.

Grand Rounds were received hesitantly at first, due to the staff's feelings of inadequacy in presenting formal issues. When Jane made them realize the simplest of issues could be presented, such as diabetic foot care, this sparked an interest to discuss grand round topics. Jane also provided use of audiovisual equipment, photocopying privileges for hand-outs, and the use of the boardroom for presentations. This created an aura of prestige for grand rounds and contributed to both the acceptance of rounds and to the professionalism of being a nurse. Jane felt hopeful that this professionalism would promote the quality care she wanted at University Hospital.

The *Patient Questionnaire Mechanism* was designed by the staff on 4 East. The staff felt the objectives in utilizing this quality assurance tool were twofold. The one drawback to such a questionnaire can be bias; therefore, both a concurrent and a retrospective questionnaire would be requested from each patient. The second objective was to keep the questionnaire short, clear, and measurable. Jane's premise was that the staff would benefit most from this tool if they monitored distribution and collection of the data. Jane's role would be to help interpret the data, assist in providing resolutions to any problems presented, and provide feedback to administration. The overall feeling both the staff and Jane had about patient questionnaires was that the use of this tool was limited and should always be correlated with other quality assurance programs.

The professional role expansion included all of the above ways of contributing to quality care. In addition, Jane wanted her staff to know that she actively believed in professional nursing, and that she would promote it. A few of the ways she demonstrated this was first to allow each professional nurse three conference days a year to attend outside workshops or seminars. The staff was expected to present their workship seminar notes. Jane made sure time would be allocated on the monthly schedule for such presentations. Jane also encouraged participation in ANA and NLN meetings and activities, and on occasion she and the staff worked out a carpool to such functions.

Scheduling was the third major area Jane felt needed to be shared with the staff. Since scheduling can often be viewed as a weapon administration has over staff, Jane wanted to set guidelines by which the staff could prepare their own schedules. For example, guidelines could include items such as:

1. Each shift has to be covered with the appropriate type and number of personnel.
2. Everyone has equal weekends and late shifts off.
3. Each member needs to coordinate conference days or requested days off so as not to conflict.

In conclusion, one could see Jane's ideas of optimal quality care were promoted through such programs as audits, rounds, questionnaires, and active professional encouragement.

Over coffee the next day, Fran was asked how she could promote quality care. She responded, "I believe that the staff workers, by having as much autonomy as possible, can truly provide the quality of care wanted by hospital administration; but personnel need to be involved and included. Quality needs to be instilled, not commanded of people. Development of nursing quality assurance needs motivational ideas in the forefront of planning."

"Education of the Nurse Manager and staff needs

*to be a priority. I need to always function as a Role
Model. . . ."*

Staff Development

Fran knew that there were many new staff members
arriving on her unit. She was very aware that these
new people needed not only much support and encouragement, but that they had to be fully functional
within a short period of time.

Fran contacted *the Staff Development Department,*
and asked Ms. Sally Brightlights if she could meet
with her for lunch.

Ms. Brightlights arrived wearing a crisp white uni-
form and sparkling white shoes. While getting her
salad, Fran thought . . . "She really looks the role of
the nurse practicing at the bedside."

Fran asked Sally Brightlights, "Just what will you
teach the new orientees?" "Oh, what they need to
know," Sally replied. "It really is very simple."

Sally then went on to describe her orientation program. *"Orientation is an important function of a Staff
Development Department.* I not only teach the new
employees our *Standards,* but I try to help them *know
where they should go if they have any questions."*

"Recently," Sally said, "we have developed *Self-
Learning Modules.* The student can *learn at his or her
own leisure,* complete tests to recognize the knowledge gained, and move on from there.".

"That is a whole new idea," thought Fran. *"Everyone does learn in different time frames."* Sally said,
"Orientation is only as good as the positive reinforcement and the support you provide on the nursing
unit."

Sally suggested that Fran identify *Preceptors* for the

new employees. A *Preceptor* should be available on a one-to-one basis for the new person. That preceptor becomes the *Role Model*. She informs, demonstrates procedures, and supports the new person.

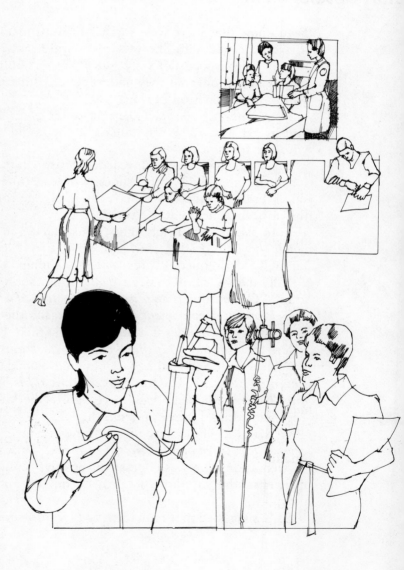

Fran began to discuss who among her competent staff could function as role models. By dessert time, she had identified preceptors for all of her new staff.

Suddenly Sally asked, "Fran, are you going to the Continuing Educational Program that is being sponsored by our hospital? Did you know that we are going to have the opportunity to hear and meet Dr. National Nursing Leader from California?"

"Well," said Fran, "I saw the flyer, but I was not sure if the topic pertained to my floor." "Oh, yes," said Sally. "You know these Continuing Educational Programs can provide for all of us. Not only will this program meet the requirements for our licensure update, but we will also be exposed to a leader in nursing who could *expand our horizons.*" "Well," Fran thought, "Staff Development has two functions . . . Sally Brightlights is responsible for not only coordinating *Orientation,* but also for planning *Continuing Education.*" Unconsciously, Fran had spoken out loud, and Sally, with a twinkle in her eye, said, "Oh, our Department does even more. We have *responsibility for ensuring that staff has the knowledge base to perform safely.* Do you know about our *Roving Road Shows?*" "Oh yes," said Fran. "That is when you come on the unit and do a *Show and Tell* about a certain piece of equipment."

Sally said, "I also attend many meetings. One of them is the Products and Procedure Committee Meeting. I am very aware that when a new piece of equipment is bought, staff members need to be instructed on how to use it safely."

"So," said Fran. "You really have three important functions."

Orientation
Continuing Education
Inservice education

"Yes," said Sally Brightlights " . . . Our role is vital, and our responsibility is *to teach* and *to coach* those staff who lack knowledge to perform on the job."

"Well," said Fran. "Your job is very important . . . you are a valuable *Support to us.* Don't worry, I will keep in touch, and we will use your Department in helping us to stay current and to provide safe practice."

Performance Evaluation

Fran knew that part of her responsibility as a nurse manager was to let her *employees know where they have been, where they are now, and where they are going in the future.* She also needed time with the employees to share *her Goals,* and *the Goals of the Institution.*

Her Director of Nursing had formed a committee and that committee had developed *Competency-Based Job Descriptions.* These criteria greatly helped Fran because they reduced personal bias in the evaluation of her staff.

The *Criteria* established by the committee *allowed the staff to advance through a Career Ladder.* The *Career Ladder provided a Mechanism for Clinical Promotion.* (Shride, 1982). It could be used to reward a nurse for clinical competence, knowledge, and performance (Shride, 1982). Of course, movement to an upward rung on the ladder was accompanied by a monetary reward.

This competency-based career ladder forced Fran to observe and scrutinize the work of her employees. She made a point of observing all aspects of an em-

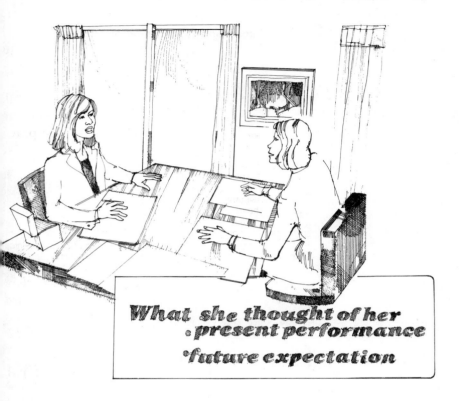

ploye's job at different times and on different days (Metzger, 1978, p. 45).

Setting the Stage

Fran always gave her employees advance notice of an upcoming evaluation. In that notice, she requested that the employee do a *Self-Evaluation*. A Self-Evaluation could assist Fran in determining where the employee thought she or he really was. Fran also made sure that the employee knew the promotion process

Career Ladders for the Registered Nurse

Administrative
track

Level V	Division director				
Level IV	Head nurse				
Level III	Assistant head nurse				
Staff nurse*	Clinician I	Clinician II	Clinician III	Clinical nurse specialist	Clinical track
	Level II	Level III	Level IV	Level V	

*Entry level — staff nurse

at the hospital and how to advance through the ladder.

Getting Started

The evaluation was always done in private with minimum interruptions.

The conference always started on *a friendly note.* Fran then asked the employee what the employee thought of his or her job, present performance, and expectations for the future.

Planning Productively

Fran and the employee mutually planned goals and objectives. Fran always started with an *Action Verb*

University Hospital Nursing Department: Comparison of Assessment Skills Expected at RN Level, Clinician I Level, and Clinician II Level

Clinical Position	Evaluation Score*					

Registered Nurse

Assessment

1. Assesses patient and family needs and completes admission assessment documentation — 1 2 3 4 5 NA

2. Compiles and maintains a problem list from assessment information on Nursing Care Plan — 1 2 3 4 5 NA

Clinician I

Assessment

1. Identifies physical, social, and psychosocial needs of the patient and his family — 1 2 3 4 5 NA

2. Performs physical assessment
   a Records data on admission nursing assessment form — 1 2 3 4 5 NA
   b Recognizes and calls attention to subtle physiologic changes in the patient — 1 2 3 4 5 NA

3. Identifies pertinent diagnostic data and reports and records them — 1 2 3 4 5 NA

Clinician II

Assessment

1. Performs nursing assessment and obtains patient health history, utilizing information from the — 1 2 3 4 5 NA

(Continued)

University Hospital Nursing Department: Comparison of Assessment Skills Expected at RN Level, Clinician I Level, and Clinician II Level (*Continued*)

Clinical Position	Evaluation Score*
patient, family, chart, other nurses, community agencies, professional staff, and other hospital departments	
2. Identifies immediate and long-term physical, social, and psychological needs of the patient and family and sets priorities related to these needs	1 2 3 4 5 NA
3. Records and reports pertinent data on the patient's record and to appropriate health-care team members	1 2 3 4 5 NA
4. Follows diagnostic data closely, discriminating between normal/abnormal values and their effect on the patient's progress and/or recovery	1 2 3 4 5 NA
5. Determines which nursing situations require immediate action and responds accordingly	1 2 3 4 5 NA
6. Identifies patient's support systems	1 2 3 4 5 NA

(Shride S: Competency Based Career Ladder. Cabell Huntington Hospital, West Virginia, 1982)
*Evaluation scoring: 1 = exceeds standard;
            3 = meets standards consistently;
            5 = never meets standards

like: "We need to *Implement* Primary Nursing Care within six months." She was always *Consistent* and made sure only one idea was expressed at a time.

Fran knew that the number-one motivator of people is *Feedback* on *Results* (Blanchard and Johnson, 1982, p. 87). Fran made unit rounds frequently over the year, and whenever she saw a positive or a negative action, she quickly complimented or commented on the behavior. She never attacked a person's worth or value as a person, she only reprimanded the behavior (Blanchard and Johnson, 1982, p. 55).

Ending the Performance Evaluation Process

Fran always concluded the conference with an overall objective for the employee. This objective could *always be attained* if the *employee functioned satisfactorily.* Her *Goal* was to develop *Champions,* and in order to *develop a Champion . . . one had to Achieve and Succeed.*

Fran always asked the employee:

"Do you want to achieve?"
"How will you achieve?"
"When will you do it?"
"How will you get it done?"

Fran always made sure employees knew the goals of the organization. She hoped that they believed in these goals, and, *best of all, the employees always left the evaluation conference* with a *full knowledge of*

WHAT THEIR NURSE MANAGER EXPECTS OF THEM . . . AND WHAT THE EMPLOYEE COULD EXPECT OF THE NURSE MANAGER . . . .

And always, Fran would plan another meeting . . . just for *Follow-up.*

Collective Bargaining*

It had been a very busy morning, and as the day progressed, Murphy's Law was in full swing. Everything that could go wrong, did. Consequently, Fran was late for lunch. She had missed her co-workers and was eating alone. She sighed deeply and took a small bite from her sandwich. Her ears perked up as she heard the words "union" and "collective bargaining" from the group of nurses who were lunching at a nearby table.

As these nurses continued their discussion, in whispered tones with their heads close together, several things emerged: the nurses were unhappy in their present work situation; they did not think the existing administrative structure was responsive to their concerns; and methods used in the past had not been effective in bringing about change. Later in the discussion, the nurses expressed other feelings: they were being overworked; there were not enough nurses on each unit; there were too many hours of overtime; they were unable to gain appointments to decision-making committees; they were working on a salary scale at least 10 percent lower than the staff nurses in other area hospitals; and they were not receiving tuition support to further their education.

Fran was disturbed about some of the same issues but the thought of collective bargaining made her feel anxious and more than a little uncomfortable. She thought to herself, "There must be other options, but I really need to know more about collective bargaining before I decide that it is not viable just because it makes me feel uncomfortable."

After several trips to the library and an in-depth

*Contributed by Dr. Rita Sellers

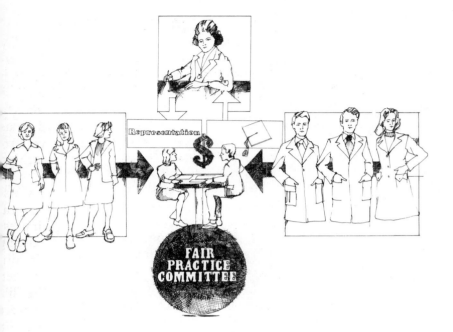

research of the literature regarding collective bargaining and nursing, Fran became better informed. She learned that nurses' concerns with their work situation were not unlike those of teachers, university professors, and other professional workers. Moreover, she discovered that *collective bargaining was initiated by laborers as early as* 1636. At that time, it was spurned by professional workers. *They were preoccupied with the development of their individual professions.*

The 1960s and 1970s saw tremendous increases in professional workers' involvement in collective bargaining. The movement was lead by public school teachers, who were joined by college professors, social workers, and others.

The majority of nurses *were excluded* from the *col-*

lective bargaining process by an amendment to the *National Labor Relations Act* that exempted charitable hospitals from the law. Consequently, it was not until 1974, when the *Taft Hartley Act* was amended, bringing nurses and other health workers in hospitals and nursing homes under the jurisdiction of the National Labor Relations Board, that the *nurses were in a position to demand that the hospital administration bargain with them collectively.*

As Fran explored the situation in her hospital, she tried very hard to understand the nature of the problem and how she could become part of the solution. She learned that in those institutions where open, free flowing channels of communication existed between the staff nurses and the administration, there was no talk of collective bargaining.

If the staff nurses decided to pursue collective bargaining, there were some *clearly identified guidelines* she, as a part of the administration, must follow. The Administration must ensure free choice of representation to its employees. As a *Nurse Manager*, Fran was *part of the Hospital Administration;* therefore she was *not free to influence the staff nurses in their voting for or against collective bargaining.* It is also the responsibility of Administration to *arrange for each employee to cast a secret ballot in an election supervised by the National Labor Relations Board* (Boyer, Westerhaus, and Coggeshall, 1975, p. 177). So, Fran, as a Nurse Manager, would have to make it possible for her staff to vote their desires.

Many of her staff nurses, as they had done in the past, came to Fran for direction. She reminded them of how one uses the problem-solving process:

Identifying the problem
Collecting and analyzing data

Developing and implementing a plan
Evaluating its effectiveness

As the staff nurses applied this process to their concerns, they were able to clarify the problems and identify a number of options as potential solutions. The nurses proceeded to work among themselves, and Fran began to use the problem-solving process at her level.

At the next Administrative Staff Meeting, she voiced her concerns about the staff nurses' low salary schedules and lack of representation on decision-making committees, and how these tended to lower the standards of patient care. She found to her dismay that she was not alone. A number of the administrators shared her concerns, and they were able to identify other concerns of equal value that deserved consideration. As a result of the meeting, a committee from the administrative staff met with the hospital administrator to share these concerns. The serendipity of the timing was very fortuitous because the hospital administrator was in the process of developing the budget for the next fiscal year and could make some immediate changes in the salary schedules. The hospital was also developing a long-range plan and was therefore able to plan for a number of other changes in the work situation of the nurses in a structured, thoughtful manner.

Two months later at the Administrative Staff Meeting, the Director of Nursing reported that the subcommittee of the Administrative Staff had been very helpful in providing support for change in several hospital policies. As a result, plans were underway for the following: an 8 percent raise for the entire nursing staff effective at the beginning of the next fiscal year (fifteen days away); an increase of 70 percent in the monies provided for continuing education and a change in the policy to include tuition reimbursement; a feasibility plan for a daycare center for preschool and school-age children under the age of twelve; a choice of HMO or Blue Cross and Blue Shield as illness insurance (rather than just Blue Cross and Blue Shield) and a feasibility plan to develop a Joint Practice Committee with a rotating chairperson. The Joint Practice Committee would have representation from the various departments of Nursing and Medicine, and the role of chairperson would rotate at six-month intervals.

As Fran mused over the events of the last two months, she was again impressed with what appropriate leadership could accomplish. She had approached a problem thoughtfully and had involved her co-workers in tackling the identified problem, and this team approach had yielded results. The staff nurses were much happier in their work situation, the level of care for patients was continuing to improve, and, with more nurses increasing their education, nursing care would get even better. But the issue that pleased Fran most was the plan to establish a Joint Practice Committee. The idea of a structured forum that supported nurses and physicians, sitting down as colleagues to work out their common concerns about patient care, was truly exhilarating.

Patient Classification Systems

The number of nurses needed to provide care on Fran's unit was not consistent. On some days, Fran's staff had fewer patients, yet more professional registered nurses were needed. On other days, there were more

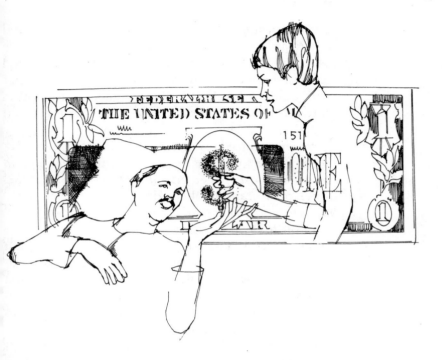

patients, yet fewer staff members were needed. Problems surfaced when her census was down. The nursing office would call and request that the nurses float to other units. It was on just those days that the bottom would fall out of the unit.

Fran believed that staffing a floor based simply on the number of beds filled did not address the real requirements of patients. Some patients only needed two hours of care in a twenty-four-hour period, while other patients truly needed ten hours of care.

Her hospital was being reimbursed only for a specific amount per patient stay, depending on the patient's diagnosis. All of the other services in the hospital could quantify and qualify their costs. She was also convinced that *the service the nurse gave was a tangible product.* She felt that the services rendered to patients could be measured in terms of patient care needs. If these needs required that the nurse spend certain amounts of time with her patients, then that time could have a dollar value assigned to it. In other words, *the cost of nursing care* could be *priced out in dollars and cents.*

Fran introduced the idea at a nursing administrative meeting. She knew that she needed the *blessing and overall support* of her *Nursing Director.* She stated in her presentation: "Itemizing Nursing Care is *the only sensible business-like approach to getting a firm grasp on the true costs of care.*"

The Director of Nursing said that she would consult with Hospital Administration. The Director said that many departments would be involved in the selection of a company that could provide the consultation services, as well as software and hardware needed to implement a computerized system.

A month later, Fran was invited to become part of a committee that would review Patient Classification Systems.

The committee recommended that a computer system be purchased that would enable the nurse managers to respond effectively to the changing status of patients, would control resources in the face of rising costs, and would meet Joint Commission on Accreditation of Hospitals Standards. Fran suggested to the committee that she, as a Nurse Manager, needed the following information on a daily basis:

Professional/nonprofessional staffing needs

Percent occupancy on the unit

Average patient type

Nursing care hours for the unit

The hours per patient day

The total number of personnel required for
twenty-four hours

A method of tracking costs of nursing care per
patient and per nursing unit

The committee members all agreed that this system
had to relate workload with quality of care. They also
agreed that the daily reports had to be easy to read.
All felt that the information had to be provided not
two weeks later, but on the *same date.*

Many companies were contacted. It was an exciting
day when one vendor O'Leary and Associates, Inc.
was selected to work with the Department to institute
a nursing management information system. The Consulting Firm, as well as the Director of Nursing, agreed
on an implementation approach to classify patients.

A *Coordinating Committee* was selected, which
consisted of individuals who would provide maximum representation throughout the agency. Some of
the members of this committee were the Comptroller,
the Hospital Administrator, the Director of Nursing,
and the Systems Analyst. They would meet only once
every six weeks. Their purpose was to review the status and to approve the workings of the Working Committee.

The Working Committee, which would meet weekly,
would consist of all those who could best assess the
patient care needs on their nursing units. This committee consisted of Nurse Managers and staff nurses
from all three shifts.

The system that was adopted categorized the patients according to an assessment of their nursing care
requirements over a specified period of time. It evaluated the patients':

Biophysiologic needs
Psychosocial needs
Educational needs
Procedural needs

The Working Committee met with the Consultants and reviewed existing definitions. They revised those that were needed in order to individualize the system to the hospital.

The following are examples of the approved definitions:

Admission/Discharge:

Mark in pencil if patient has arrived or will arrive by 6:00 PM. Mark if patient discharged or transferred from unit or within unit during shift. Includes death.

Indicator:

One-to-One Restriction. Place a mark if the patient requires constant nurse supervision, *e.g.,* Suicide Risk. If this indicator is checked, do not check any other indicators.

Feed, Partial Assist:

Mark if patient requires assistance to eat. Include opening, positioning of cartons, silverware, etc. Isolation.

FORM - 3/4 GLOBE 458676-0

	Row										
Unit	40	0	1	2	3	4	5	6	7	8	9
	39										
DRG:	38	0	1	2	3	4	5	6	7	8	9
	37										
	36	0	1	2	3	4	5	6	7	8	9
PATIENT NO:	35										
	34	0	1	2	3	4	5	6	7	8	9
	33										
	32	0	1	2	3	4	5	6	7	8	9
	31										
	30	0	1	2	3	4	5	6	7	8	9
	29										
	28	0	1	2	3	4	5	6	7	8	9

- [ ] Admission / Discharge
- [ ] Indicator
- [ ] Feed — Partial Assist.
- [ ] Feed — Total Assist.
- [ ] Fluid & Elect. Class 1
- [ ] Fluid & Elect. Class 2
- [ ] Fluid & Elect. Class 3
- [ ] Elimination - Simple
- [ ] Elimination - Complex
- [ ] Wound Care — Simple
- [ ] Wound Care — Complex
- [ ] Tube Care
- [ ] Pulmonary — 1
- [ ] Pulmonary — 2
- [ ] Physical Activity - Partial
- [ ] Physical Activity - Total
- [ ] Special Needs
- [ ] Physical Protection
- [ ] Assess Complex
- [ ] Special Emotional Needs
- [ ] Learning Needs — Simple
- [ ] Learning Needs — Complex
- [ ] Surgical Proc. & Testing
- [ ] Support — 1
- [ ] Support — 2
- [ ] Support — 3
- [ ] Qualifier

There were twenty-four indicators, and once these were checked on the card in pencil, the card could easily be fed into a card reader. The computer calculated the indicators and identified the exact number of professional and nonprofessional staff needed.

The Working Committee also developed an orientation booklet that defined the rules of the system. Some of the standards discussed were:

Who should classify? . . . Only the Registered Nurse caring for the patient.

Which shift should classify? . . . In most situations, once a day at 9 AM.

The Consultants provided extensive educational programs for all of those in the Department. They informed the Registered Nurses that they were only to *mark those indicators that applied to a patient.* The Consultants also taught the Unit Secretaries how to fill in the DRG Number, the Patient Number, and the Unit Number. It was an exciting day when the hospital purchased the microcomputer, software, card reader, and printer.

Fran's unit was the first unit to start classifying their patients. The staff mambers were all amazed that when they classified their patients at 9 AM, the report was generated by 9:30 AM.

The system also provided staffing cards, and, when those were fed into the computer, a comparison report was generated. This report was most helpful in determining whether or not the nursing staff was over- or underutilized.

The entire nursing department now had a management tool, a patient classification system, that enabled the entire department to effectively manage the allocation of human resources. The number of people

HOSPITAL MEDICAL CENTER

NURSING SERVICE DEPARTMENT

PATIENT CLASSIFICATION SYSTEM

MED. / SURG.   CENSUS 34 PATIENTS

DATE   02/21/86   CAPACITY 37 BEDS

    PATIENT TYPE :

       TYPE I   7

       TYPE II   15   PERCENT OCCUPANCY   91.8 %

       TYPE III   7

       TYPE IV   5

       TYPE V   0   AVERAGE PAT. TYPE = 2.29

       TYPE VI   0

TOTAL CENSUS =   34

TOTAL REQUIRED NURSING CARE HOURS = 183

HOURS PER PATIENT DAY OR HPPD = 5.3

REQUIRED PERSONNEL FOR DIRECT 24 HOUR CARE = 22.8
              UNIT CONSTANT (HEAD NURSE) =   1.0

              TOTAL PERSONNEL FOR 24 HOURS = 23.8

PERSONNEL DISTRIBUTION PER SHIFT   PERSONNEL MIX
---------------------------------   -------------

    DAYS =   10.2   PROFESSIONAL(RN)   60 %

    EVENINGS = 7.9   NON PROFESSIONAL   40 %

    NIGHTS =   5.7

    PERSONNEL BREAKDOWN BY SHIFT PER 24 HOURS.

    DAYS   6.12 R.N.   4.08 LGPN, TECH OR NA

    EVENINGS   4.74 R.N.   3.16 LGPN, TECH OR NA

    NIGHTS   3.42 R.N.   2.28 LGPN, TECH OR NA

    THE HEAD NURSE IS NOT INCLUDED IN THE ABOVE DISTRIBUTION OR MIX.

NURSING SERVICE DEPARTMENT

HOSPITAL STAFFING REPORT

DATE 02/21/86

UNIT	PATIENTS	PERSONNEL MIX NEEDED			PERSONNEL MIX ACTUAL		UNIT STATISTICS
		PROF.	NON-P.	TOTAL	PROF.	NON-P.	CENSUS = 66
	TYPE I = 12						H.P.P.D. = 8.1
	TYPE II = 23						
	TYPE III = 15	DA = 19.5	DA = 7	= 26.5	DA = 20	DA = 8	OCCUPANCY= 81.4%
81 BEDS	TYPE IV = 16	EV = 15.5	EV = 4.9	= 20.3	EV = 16	EV = 5	A.P.T. = 2.5
	TYPE V = 0	NI = 14.6	NI = 4.1	= 18.7	NI = 15	NI = 4	N CARE HR= 543
	TYPE VI = 0	TOT= 49.6	TOT= 16	= 65.5	TOT= 51	TOT= 17	REQ PER = 65.5
							ACT PER = 68

	PROFESSIONAL			NON-PROFESSIONAL			TOTAL STAFF		
	ACTUAL	REQ'D	DIFF.	ACTUAL	REQ'D	DIFF.	ACTUAL	REQ'D	DIFF.
	DA = 20	19.5	.5	DA = 8	7	1	DA = 28	26.5	1.5
SUMMARY	EV = 16	15.5	.5	EV = 5	4.9	0	EV = 21	20.3	.7
	NI = 15	14.6	.3	NI = 4	4.1	-.1	NI = 19	18.7	.2
	TOT= 51	49.6	1.4	TOT= 17	16	1	TOT= 68	65.5	2.5

* *

needed to care for patients could now be met. The nursing department now met the standards of Joint Commission on Accreditation of Hospitals and they also had a firm grasp on the true costs of care.

The patient classification system was implemented in less than six months. This information was most helpful to Fran, for she now had information that increased her ability, as a manager, to determine her staffing requirements.

The Implementation of Professional Delivery Systems

One particular Thursday, the entire nursing floor was in chaos. The Team Leaders ran from 7 AM until 4 PM. All of the staff just seemed to be providing crisis care to their patients. The medication nurse gave a patient the wrong medication. Someone left siderails down on a confused patient, and the patient fell out of bed. One of the patients being discharged really did not know how to care for his diabetes . . . . It was one of those days when Fran almost wished she had rolled over in bed and continued to sleep through the day.

During this hectic time, Fran supported her staff and assisted in providing care wherever necessary. Although frustrated, she knew that she had to give support in order to help her staff just *make it through the day.*

While driving home, Fran began to be objective about some of the problem. She thought, "The staff on 5 West is forced to provide care for too many people at one time. It is almost like too much electricity; the more the voltage, the higher and higher the emotional overload. It's like a wire with too much electricity flowing through it. Eventually the nurses will burn out and disconnect."

Fran had been reading about *Primary Nursing and the creation of Professional Practice Environment.* Her research took her to a description of the *Case Mo-*

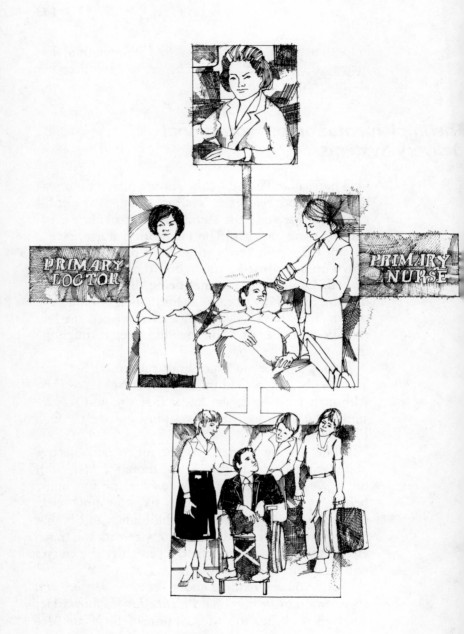

PRIMARY
DOCTOR

PRIMARY
NURSE

dality of Care. The case modality was similar to the private duty nursing concept. In this situation, one nurse provided total patient care.

The *Functional Modality* originated as a task-oriented system, whereby divisions of labor were viewed apart from patient needs. It was thought that if Henry Ford could develop an automobile by utilizing functional assignments to complete a task, why could not nursing. In this situation, one nurse administered medications, another provided treatments, and others bathed patients. Tasks became the top priority—the method of achieving satisfactory outcomes for patients. Patients exposed to this type of nursing saw many caretakers, but no one in particular was significant in their care. Goals for patients were often never defined, and the emphasis by nursing was placed on quantity rather than quality.

Fran's unit had been functioning on the Team Modality during that crisis day. Why? Well, it was the accepted care modality at the hospital. Her thirty-nine-bed medical/surgical unit staff was broken into two teams. The best-prepared nurses became the Team Leaders. It was the Team Leader's responsibility to prepare the assignments, to dispense medications and treatments, and to supervise the direct care of about twenty patients. Often these dedicated team leaders barely saw their patients, let alone completed their care plans . . . that is, unless the Joint Commission on Accreditation of Hospitals was going to visit the hospital.

Fran reviewed articles about Primary Nursing and saw that this system was similar to the Case Method on which nursing was first established. Primary Nursing allows autonomous practitioners to have a direct line of access to patients. Each nurse in the Primary Nursing Care System was responsible for the total nursing care of her patients for the twenty-four-hour period. The case load ranged from one or two patients in intensive care to six to eight patients on a regular medical/surgical unit. The Primary Nurse, who functioned either on the day shift or the evening shift, defined the care requirements and delegated these responsibilities to an Associate Nurse. The Primary Nurse could clearly identify herself to her patients, often with a calling card that read:

HELLO! I am your Primary Nurse.

My Name Is:

_____ R.N.

Each Primary Nurse could establish a contract with her patients from the time of admission to discharge from the hospital. The Primary Nurse was totally responsible for planning the total patient care during the hospitalization. She could learn to interact and communicate effectively with the Associate Nurses, the Physicians, the family unit, and the hospital departments. She could accept total responsibility for the care and follow-through for her patients. This system could allow autonomous practitioners to have a direct line of access to patients. It was different from the other systems, such as the functional and team method, in that it could result in increased responsibility and autonomy.

Nursing Process

The nursing process could certainly become more meaningful, for the assessment could lead to the identification of patient problems (Nursing Diagnosis) and the development of necessary solutions. These solutions, once placed on the care plan, are then implemented (The Doing). The Primary Nurse could then assess if the goals were accomplished (Evaluation).

This system certainly could broaden the nurses responsibility, and with this broadened responsibility could come autonomy. Fran thought, "Autonomy for nursing means the ability to make decisions *with* the patient. It means mutual access between the patient and practitioners without the *Nurse Manager* or the Director of Nursing acting as the gate keeper of services. Autonomy means *that the nurse can and will provide nursing care directly to patients.* In this system, nurses can be responsible for their own practice decisions, and they can be accountable to their patients."

Fran envisioned that if primary nursing was im-

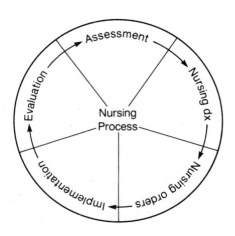

plemented, then the nurse could directly know the *Diagnostic Related Groupings* of her patients and could be responsible for monitoring each patient's entire length of stay. If the first-line caretaker could have full responsibility for the patient length of stay, the patients might be discharged earlier. This *Prepared Discharge Process* could save the hospital millions of dollars . . . dollars that could be utilized for other things.

"Once the Primary Nursing Care System is in place," Fran dreamed . . . "we could evolve to a model of *Joint Practice.* In this environment, the same nurse could carry the same caseload as the primary physician. This system could promise not only to improve the working relationship between physicians and nurses, but once again would give the nurses the professional responsibility that they deserve."

Primary Nursing

Upon arriving home, Fran decided that *Primary Nursing* was the way to go. This system would eliminate burnout and provide the patients a *Quality Comprehensive Service.*

The next day Fran returned to the nursing unit and discussed her ideas with the staff. The staff, along with Fran, requested a meeting with Nursing Administration. They knew that they needed support all the way from the top of the organization.

The Director of Nursing believed in this philosophy and requested a plan for implementation from the nursing unit. At the same time, the Director of Nursing said that she would meet with the Executive Committee of the Hospital, as well as inform the medical staff and the Board of Trustees. She also said that there were many support systems (consultants) available to provide all of the necessary education and training to implement the system. A few months later, after approval from the Board of Trustees, and with support from the Medical Staff and Hospital Administration, a consultant conducted hospital-wide educational programs. The pilot unit was identified as 5 West.

The entire nursing staff on the unit participated in rewriting their job descriptions. The nursing unit consisted of thirty-nine beds. The staff decided that they would adopt the district method of primary nursing. That meant that specific geographic areas on the floor were delineated into sections.

There were primary nurses identified on the day shift and others identified on the evening shift. Two districts shared the medication cart. The charts were decentralized and placed outside the patients' doors. This decentralization of the charting system enabled the primary and associate nurses to chart pertinent observations by patient. The Primary Nurse's name was identified side by side with the primary physician's name.

Districts were also identified by boards that delin-

*District number
†Number of patients

District #	Room #	MD	Primary RN	Associate RN
1	360	Smith	Hapen	Jones
	361	Smith	Hapen	Jones
	362	Smith	Hapen	Jones

eated district number, physicians, patient room number, and the name of the primary and associate nurses.

These boards helped visitors, physicians, and staff locate the nurses, who would now spend much of their time in the patients' rooms.

Change of Shift Report

In the past, the staff had utilized the tape shift reporting system and were dissatisfied with this system. Often the tape was made one or two hours before the change of shift. After the shift report, those responsible for care often found the status or condition of the patient dramatically altered.

The staff decided, as a group, to institute walking rounds. They defined this as a *Client-Centered Method of Reporting*. The Primary Nurse and the Associate Nurse would walk into the room and involve the patient in the total review of the activities of the day. During this time, the Primary Nurse would define problems of care for the Associate Nurse, as well as needed solutions. The patients began to participate in their care and gained a greater knowledge of what was happening.

Fran participated in frequent rounds during the day. In this manner, she kept abreast of the status of the nursing unit. Clinical Rounds were often conducted by the staff, and the environment became one of motivated practitioners continually seeking new knowledge.

Outcomes

A year later, Fran reflected back on the trying days of Team Nursing. Staff were now leaving the unit on time, there were fewer errors, and morale was very high. Her nurses had achieved autonomy . . . accountability . . . and now the program of Primary Nursing was evolving to that of *Joint Practice*. The staff was interacting and communicating effectively with physicians. The nurses were accepting the total responsibility for this care and follow-through.

The patients were favorably impressed with being cared for by one nurse. The patients sensed a genuine concern for them as persons, and often when rehospitalized they requested a return to the same nursing care unit.

The nurses became the *Advocates* for the patients. They had the *Authority,* the *Responsibility,* and all together they kept on striving to meet the demands or the needs of their patients and families.

References

Blanchard K, Johnson S: The One Minute Manager. New York, William Morrow & Co, 1982

Boyer JM, Westerhaus CL, Coggeshall JJ: Employee Relations and Collective Bargaining in Health Care Facilities. St Louis, CV Mosby, 1975

Metzger N: The Health Care Supervisor's Handbook. Germantown, MD, Aspen Systems, 1978

National League for Nursing: Developing a philosophy and objectives for a nursing department. Nursing Service News 2(1), 1980

Reilly DE: Behavioral Objectives: Evaluation in Nursing, 2nd ed. New York, Appleton-Century-Crofts, 1980

Rowland HS, Rowland BL: Hospital Administration Handbook. Rockville, MD, Aspen Systems, 1984

Shride S: Competency Based Career Ladder. Cabell Huntington Hospital, West Virginia, 1982

Stevens B: The Nurse as Executive, 2nd ed. Wakefield, MA, Nursing Resources, 1980

Warner M: Simulation presented for Villanova University Graduate Nursing Course, April, 1983

Urdang L (ed): Mosby's Medical and Nursing Dictionary. St Louis, CV Mosby, 1983

Conclusion

Ten years have passed and one day while meeting with the Chairman of the Board for lunch, Fran found herself discussing the possibility of becoming the Vice-President of Nursing at University Hospital. Joan Majors, the Vice-President, had decided to retire.

The Chairman, Successful Harry Smartweather, asked her, "Fran, how do you see yourself as a Manager?" "Well," said Fran, "I see *management in three stages* . . . . To be effective, *you must know yourself,* and know your strengths and weaknesses." "Then," nodded Fran, *"You must know the Principles of Management* and *how to Play the Game.*

She leaned forward, saying, "I know *Professional Nursing,* and I have gained that knowledge through my education, my readings, my mentors, networking, and conferences. Also, my recent appointment to President of the State Professional Organization has enabled me to further practice my management skills."

"Well," said Mr. Smartweather. "You also have worked very hard at being *visible;* you always *look the role,* and *act the role* of an Administrator. You also let people know your feelings . . . you are *assertive.* You have *set goals* with your staff and have allowed *them to achieve those goals.*"

"Well," said Fran, "You know that if the search committee chooses me as the new Vice-President, I will continue to use the same traits that helped me to move where I am in the organization. I really feel good about myself, and over these ten years, I do feel that I have achieved *self-confidence*. You know, Harry, I work hard . . . but I also take time out to play . . . and *smell the roses*. . . ."

Fran began to think out loud, "I have, in my *Second Stage,* tried very hard to learn the *Principles of Management* by reading and returning to school. I have developed *Champions* in this organization through *Perceptive Communication* with staff and through *Involvement of Groups.* I believe that people can become *motivated* by *allowing* the *workers at the front line* to feel *good about themselves.* I encouraged their *Participation* and *allowed them to become Winners and Champions.*"

"Fran," said Mr. Smartweather, "When you first came to the hospital as a staff nurse, you *always volunteered* for the extra projects . . . and *you followed through.* You knew that *change* took *time.* It amazed me to see you *involve people in* many of your *decisions.* You really made an effort to *involve people,* especially *when the decisions resulted* in staff *having to change their behavior.*"

"Somehow," he continued, "You always *knew the right people in the right places.*" And he said, with a twinkle in his eye, "You *aligned yourself to those leaders.* You *expanded your territory* by knowing the *people in the high places,* and by helping them *resolve problems.* It became very easy for those in management *to lean on you,* and to *give you more responsibility.* Once you had that responsibility, you always *seemed to be in control.*"

"Yes," said Fran, "I have always tried (but not always succeeded) *to maneuver the environment* instead of *being maneuvered,* especially during *conflict situations.* I attempt to *depersonalize conflict* by not attacking the individual, but by discussing the *activity itself.* During these times, I always tried to take extra *personal time for myself.* I'm convinced that *stress can be the downfall* of Nurse Administrators."

"I also am successful because *I manage my time effectively.*" And she said with a laugh, "This past position as the Associate Director of Nursing has been successful because I really have learned to *delegate effectively.* Once *I knew myself* and *the management principles,* I then learned *how to Play the Game.*"

"When I first arrived at the hospital, the organization was very centralized. It was because of the *leadership* of Ms. Majors that we moved to a *decentralized structure.* Believe me . . . years ago, *decisions made at the top of the organization,* because it was centralized, *never filtered down to the bottom.* Now, with *decentralization,* not only is *communication* more effective, but the *morale and enthusiasm* of the staff are great."

"Do you remember when we had an *organizing effort* from labor union 999? The staff, right in the beginning of Ms. Major's tenure, really did not believe that she could meet the needs of the staff. The reason a union doesn't exist now is mainly because Ms. Majors *restructured the organization,* and now the *Committees* within the *Nursing Organization* participate in the *Management of the Organization.* Now *decisions made at both the top and the bottom of the Organization* are known by all. There really is involvement . . . ."

"The *Patient Classification System* that I had recommended eight years ago *demonstrated* that the nursing department needed to be composed of 65 percent professional staff and 35 percent nonprofessional staff. Initially, the computer reports showed that we needed more professional staff. We increased staff and then moved the delivery system of *Team Nursing* to that of *Primary Nursing Care.* Today, our nurses really have the *autonomy and authority to make decisions with their patients.*"

"Of course, the *Staff Development Department* should get much credit in helping us during the *Implementation Phase.* They supported us through *the Change Process* as we moved from *Team* to *Primary Nursing Care.*"

"Did you know," Fran said with a smile, "The *Nursing Quality Assurance Department* recently determined that we meet our *Standards of Care* throughout the institution about 90 percent of the time?"

"Well," said Mr. Smartweather, "I hope through your direction and guidance . . . that some day, you will say to the *Board of Directors* . . . 'We now have 100 percent *compliance* to our *standards.*"

"I agree," said Fran. "I believe that we can maybe attain the *goal of 100 percent compliance* by continually encouraging and reinforcing the *development of Champions.*"

"I have much to be thankful for, Harry, . . . the *Mentors that I have had* have allowed me to *feel excited about myself.* You have also been a mentor to me, Harry; somehow, you always took the time to *support and encourage me.*"

"I see our time is up," said Harry. "I know that the search committee is very much *looking forward to meeting with you* . . . . I'll bet that they will be most impressed with your discussion of *Management in Three Stages.*"

Author Index

Angel G, Petronko DK: Developing the New Assertive Nurse: Essentials for Advancement. New York, Springer Publishing, 1983, *32*

Bailey JT, Hendricks DE: Decisions, decisions: Guidelines for making them more easily. Nursing Life 2(4):45–47, 1982, *78*

Bass BM (ed): Stogdill's Handbook of Leadership. New York, The Free Press, 1981, *20, 50, 54, 61, 68*

Blanchard K, Johnson S: The One Minute Manager. New York, William Morrow & Co, 1982, *51, 52, 53, 129*

Boyer JM, Westerhaus CL, Coggeshall JJ: Employee Relations and Collective Bargaining in Health Care Facilities. St Louis, CV Mosby, 1975, *132*

Dillon A: Reducing your stress. Nursing Life 3(3):17–24, 1982, *72*

Douglass LM: The Effective Nurse: Leader and Manager, 2nd ed. St Louis, CV Mosby, 1984, *81–82*

Korda M: Power, How to Get It, How to Use It. New York, Random House, 1975, *45*

Metzger N: The Health Care Supervisor's Handbook. Germantown, MD, Aspen Systems, 1978, *125*

National League for Nursing: Developing a philosophy and objectives for a nursing department. Nursing Service News 2(1), 1980, *106*

Newman WH, Summer CE: The Process of Management. Englewood Cliffs, NJ, Prentice-Hall, 1964, *77*

Reilly DE: Behavioral Objectives: Evaluation in Nursing, 2nd ed. New York, Appleton-Century-Crofts, 1980, *108*

Rogers C: Client Centered Therapy. Boston, Houghton Mifflin, 1965, *44*

Rowland HS, Rowland BL: Hospital Administration Handbook. Rockville, MD, Aspen Systems, 1984, *101*

Schneider S: Curing burnout while you work. Nursing Life 2(5):38–43, 1982, *73*

Shride S: Competency Based Career Ladder. Cabell Huntington Hospital, West Virginia, 1982, *123, 124, 128*

Stevens B: The Nurse as Executive, 2nd ed. Wakefield, MA, Nursing Resources, 1980, *19, 22, 105*

Tappen RM: Nursing Leadership: Concepts and Practice. Philadelphia, FA Davis, 1983, *24, 57, 58, 60*

Urdang L (ed): Mosby's Medical and Nursing Dictionary. St Louis, CV Mosby, 1983, *115*

Vance CN: The mentor connection. The Journal of Nursing Administration 12(4):7–13, 1982, *91*

Warner M: Simulation presented for Villanova University Graduate Nursing Course, April, 1983, *107*

Woodhouse DK: Change. In Marriner A (ed): Contemporary Nursing Management: Issues and Practice, pp. 302–307. St Louis, CV Mosby, 1982, *56*

Subject Index

Active medical staff, 103
Activity time sheet, 87
Associate medical staff, 103
Agendas, 46–47
Assertiveness, 30–33
Autocratic leadership style, 22

Board of Trustees, 99, 101, 103
Bureaucratic leadership style, 22

Career ladder, 123
Centralized systems, 109–110
Change, principles of, 55–61
Change agent, 55–56, 60
Chief of staff, 102–103
Chief resident responsibilities, 103–104
Collective bargaining, 130–134
Communication, perceptive, 39–43

DATE DUE

DE 28 '9 1990			
MAR 2 2 1992			
JE 13 '92			
JY 5 '92			
JY 28 '92			
FEB 2 0 1995			
11/28			
APR 0 8 1997			
NOV 1			

DEMCO 38-297